THE CANADIAN

Allergy
and Asthma

Revised
&
Updated

HANDBOOK

THE CANADIAN

Allergy *and* Asthma

Revised & Updated

HANDBOOK

by Canadian Allergists

Dr. Barry Zimmerman, MD, FRCP • Dr. Milton Gold, MD, FRCP
Dr. Sasson Lavi, MD, FRCP • Dr. Stephen Feanny, MD, FRCP

with Eleanor Brownridge, RD, FCDA

A Random House Canada / Lorraine Greey Book

A Random House Canada/Lorraine Greey Book

To the reader: This book does not presume to replace any advice from your doctor. It is intended to better enable you to work with your doctor to implement both short- and long-term strategies for treating your disease. No action should be taken solely on the information in this book, and the publisher and the authors take no responsibility for readers' actions.

Canadian Cataloguing in Publication Data

Main entry under title:

The Canadian allergy & asthma handbook

Rev. ed

Includes index.

ISBN 0–679–30790–7

1. Allergy — Popular works. 2. Asthma — Popular works. I. Zimmerman, Barry.

RC584.C35   1996   616.97   C95–932887–4

Drs. Zimmerman, Gold, Lavi and Feanny are practicing allergists in Ontario.

Published by
Random House of Canada Limited
1265 Aerowood Drive
Mississauga, Ontario L4W 1B9

Produced for Random House of Canada Limited by
Lorraine Greey Publications Limited
56 The Esplanade, Suite 303
Toronto, Ontario M5E 1A7

Designed by David Shaw and Associates Ltd.
Cover Design by Andrew Smith

Printed in Canada 12345678L32109876

Contents

About the Authors

Dr. Barry Zimmerman is the former Director of the Division of Allergy at The Hospital for Sick Children in Toronto and a member of the Asthma Centre, Toronto Hospital (Western Division).

Dr. Milton Gold is Assistant Professor of Paediatrics in the Division of Immunology/Allergy at The Hospital for Sick Children.

Dr. Sasson Lavi is staff allergist and immunologist in the Division of Immunology/Allergy at The Hospital for Sick Children.

Dr. Stephen Feanny is staff allergist and immunologist in the Division of Immunology/Allergy at The Hospital for Sick Children.

The doctors are all practicing allergists in Ontario.

Eleanor Brownridge, RD, FCDA, is a professional dietitian who regularly writes articles on nutrition and other health subjects. Her book *I'm Hungry: Your Guide to Nutritious and Tasty Food for Young Children* was published by Random House in 1987 and revised in 1993.

A Word from the Authors

In this second edition of *The Canadian Allergy and Asthma Handbook* the underlying premise for our treatment of allergies hasn't changed. More than ever, we believe that avoidance of allergens, where possible, is the best approach to allergy management. In recent years, the number of peanut-sensitive children has increased significantly. And with this life-threatening allergy, avoidance is the only safe option. With asthma, it may not be possible to avoid exposure to all allergens, such as dust mites or animal dander, but reducing the amounts in a person's environment can go a long way towards making life more enjoyable and far less stressful. Therefore, throughout this book, a major emphasis is on actions you can take to create an allergy-safe environment for yourself and others.

A recent consensus statement from Canadian allergists has urged school systems to take action to protect young children. But achieving a high level of allergy safety in schools will require a high level of awareness and cooperation from teachers, students and their parents. In nursery schools, it can mean a complete ban on peanuts and peanut butter in all children's snacks and lunches if there is one peanut-sensitive child. In elementary schools, it can mean no pets or plants in the classroom if there is a child with asthma. These small sacrifices are worth making so that a child may have a safer life. But because accidents still happen, achieving allergy safety also means training all school staff, from volunteers and caretakers to teachers and principals, on the emergency administration of adrenaline. We believe this book can help by educating not only families who are coping with allergies, but also concerned citizens who want to understand why changes are necessary and what they can do to protect the children in their care.

New drugs
In this revision we have also added new information about the medications used to treat allergies. While we don't expect patients to tell their doctors what to prescribe, we do believe that the information we are providing can help you understand why your doctor is recommending certain treatments for you and why complying with the treatment program is essential for the best results. Having read this book, allergy patients or their parents should be able to better explain their concerns to their doctors, ask appropriate questions and together develop action plans that are most suitable for the individual.

Allergy research in Canada
Historically, allergy books have described skin tests as the primary tool for diagnosis. Any person who developed areas of localized swelling soon after a small amount of pollen, food or animal material was placed under the skin was considered allergic. That person was then advised to

avoid anything that caused such swellings, and often other things as well. It meant that people labelled allergic often had a very limited lifestyle and frequently underwent marginally useful but painful treatments, such as allergy shots.

We now believe that the cause-and-effect relationship is too simplistic a way to explain all that is going on in your body, and that many of the restrictions advised by doctors and others in the past were unnecessary. Although we continue to use skin tests, we use them as just one part of our arsenal of diagnostic tools. Immediate positive skin responses do occur, but they are meaningless unless we consider the patient's symptoms and medical history along with them.

As practicing allergists, we study the scientific literature on allergy and apply it to the everyday treatment of our patients. In the twenty years we have been in practice, our patients have benefited from many exciting advances in treatment.

With this book, we'd like to acknowledge a few of our colleagues who have contributed significantly to the understanding of allergies, both in this country and throughout the world.

Dr. Jerry Dolovich of McMaster University in Hamilton has described and investigated, in a very simple and elegant way, an important phenomenon that we now call the "late response." As we mentioned, allergists historically focused on localized swellings that occurred about ten minutes after a drop of test material was placed under the skin. Dolovich observed that if this early response was a large one, it was followed by a secondary, late response several hours later. There would be an area of diffuse redness and swelling at the site, which would peak in intensity six to eight hours later. He proved that this late response was a much more complicated reaction and was based on a complex mechanism of inflammation.

Dr. Fred Hargreave, also at McMaster University in Hamilton, applied the late response theory to asthma. He proved that when airborne substances caused ongoing inflammation in the breathing tubes, the airways would become twitchy. They would go into spasm very easily. In a person with inflamed, twitchy airways, all sorts of non-specific stimuli—exercise, cold air, strong smells—could then initiate a spasm in the airways. Hargreave's concept of airway reactivity is now accepted internationally as the hallmark of asthma.

In British Columbia, Dr. Moira Chan-Yeung has applied this understanding of the nature of inflammation in the lungs to forestry workers who routinely handle western red cedar. Her studies have provided insights into how occupational exposure to substances such as grain or wood dust can cause asthma.

Despite new medications for the treatment of asthma, there is still a need to reduce exposure to certain allergens. Dr. Andrew Murray of Vancouver proved that when you reduce the number of dust mites in a person's environment, airway twitchiness is also reduced. Murray also did outstanding work proving that children with asthma have more episodes of coughing and wheezing when they are constantly being exposed to second-hand cigarette smoke.

Dr. John Toogood of London, Ontario, completed pioneer studies on the role of inhaled steroids as a way to reduce inflammation. More importantly, Toogood's studies have contributed to our understanding of the safety and possible side effects of inhaled steroids at different dosages.

The late Dr. Robert Orange of The Hospital for Sick Children in Toronto studied the changes that lead to an allergic reaction. His particular research was on the slow-reacting substances of anaphylaxis. He identified a group of body substances—called leukotrienes—that can create inflammation in airways, making it difficult to breathe.

Dr. Henry Levison, also at The Hospital for Sick Children in Toronto, taught us much about the practical understanding of the treatment of childhood asthma.

Dr. Estelle Simon of Winnipeg studied the action of antihistamines and other drug therapies used in the treatment of allergic diseases.

Today, patients in Canada and around the world are benefiting from scientifically proven, aggressive treatment plans that include both safe, efficient drug therapy and meaningful environmental changes.

We are excited about the future of allergy treatment. With major new technologies, such as genetic research, laboratory scientists are identifying exactly how genes control bodily processes. The power of these future tools is breathtaking. They will provide answers to many of the currently unresolved questions surrounding clinical allergies.

Allergies have no sexual bias; therefore, "he" and "she" are used interchangeably throughout this book.

CHAPTER ONE

Understanding Allergies

If your doctor has recently said that you or your child might have asthma or allergies, you are probably very worried about the ramifications. You may have watched with panic as your youngster sneezed and then frantically gasped for breath after petting a cat. Perhaps you've heard horror stories about people dying after eating one peanut or of someone being rushed to hospital after being stung by a bee. Maybe you've read articles in which asthma is described as a feeling of ropes wrapped so tightly around your chest that you can barely breathe, or you have friends who have turned meal preparation into a full-time chore as they try to deal with a restricted diet.

Although these and other stories are true, they are the exception. There is much unnecessary fear and hysteria about allergies. Allergy diseases are serious, but many of the complications you read or hear about are needless. If patients and their families understand more about the effective treatments available for their diseases, they can avoid most serious problems.

Just because you have allergies, it doesn't necessarily

follow that you risk having a serious reaction. Few people

> **Life-threatening allergic reactions are rare.**

with allergies are vulnerable. Many people with allergies never experience anything more severe than a mild case of eczema or occasional hay fever that responds quickly to over-the-counter medication.

In our practice, we specialize in treating children with the most difficult allergy problems. Yet if you met these children, you wouldn't know they had a disease. With modern medications, people with allergies are able to live normal, healthy lives and can participate in most activities without restriction. In fact, one out of every twelve members of the 1988 U.S. Olympic team was taking medication for asthma.

In Chapter 5, we will discuss strategies for reducing your exposure to certain things in your environment that are likely to cause problems for you. We believe this is important, but it's not the only issue. If dust is a problem,

> **A person with allergies can't change her environment completely; she must learn to live in it, and with modern medicine that is possible.**

we tell you how you can reduce the amount significantly, but no matter how carefully you clean, you can't get rid of all dust.

By combining environmental control with the other management strategies we recommend, people with asthma can sleep through the night without waking, gasping for air. They can participate in sports without coughing. Families can learn to deal with life-threatening food allergies without jeopardizing the nutritional balance of their diet or destroying their enjoyment of eating. We believe those should be the goals of treatment. Anything less compromises the quality of your life.

Allergy is a complex subject and is often misinterpreted. To protect yourself or your children, we think it helps if you understand what is going on in your own or your child's body and what your doctor is doing and recommending. We admit this can sometimes be difficult. When you visit a doctor's office, you may hear a lot of information in a short span of time; you may forget some of what was said, but reading the same advice in this book will serve as a reminder of your doctor's recommendations.

We've tried to make our explanations as simple as possible, while still ensuring that you gain an accurate picture of the process. If you do forget the meanings of some of the medical terms we use in this book, refer to the glossary on page 199.

WHAT IS AN ALLERGY?

The term **allergy** is often misused to describe any unpleasant physical reaction that can't be diagnosed otherwise. People sometimes joke about a student being "allergic to homework." The restlessness you experience after drinking coffee isn't an allergy either. It is a toxic reaction to too much caffeine; reducing your intake may be all that is needed.

> **A true allergic reaction is an inappropriate or harmful response by the immune system to normally harmless substances.**

Often parents wonder whether a child who misbehaves while at the zoo or a birthday party is allergic to the ice cream or cake. More likely this behaviour

The normal immune system

The immune system is an impressive mechanism that protects you from unfriendly elements in the environment in which you live. Every day you're exposed to myriad viruses, bacteria, parasites, fungi and other foreign substances that only occasionally invade your body and make you ill. Your immune system protects you from considerable harm or illness by destroying many of these harmful substances soon after they enter your body.

Foreign substances enter through your skin, the lining of your respiratory tract or the lining of your gastrointestinal tract. Your tissues are constantly exposed to the many substances that you touch, breathe, inhale and eat. To help protect you, the surfaces of your tissues have some natural barriers—membranes, tiny hairs and mucus secretions (phlegm). But occasionally these barriers aren't enough and foreign substances enter the tissues, either because they're very small or because there's a break in the barrier, such as a cut in your skin.

If this happens, blood rushes to the area, bringing white blood cells, which, like scavengers, engulf the foreign particle and attempt to neutralize or break it down. A specialized group of white blood cells called **lymphocytes** begins multiplying rapidly and producing compounds called **antibodies**. You can think of antibodies as spies that learn to recognize foreign particles as outsiders and remember them.

The immune response has a built-in memory. With certain infectious diseases, such as measles, you become ill only once. During your first exposure to a type of germ, your immune system makes antibodies that are specific to that unique germ. Long after you've recovered, the antibodies stay on guard in your body, ready to respond the next time that particular germ appears. Thus if you've ever had red measles, you have a storehouse of measles antibodies ready to take action the next time you encounter the red measles virus. The antibodies latch on to the foreign substance and begin a counterattack.

Antibodies can help eliminate germs in several ways. They can clump germs together so that they're easier to remove; they can kill germs directly; they can coat and neutralize poisonous substances; or they can attract other white cells that attack the germs.

The unique match between an antibody and a particular germ or foreign substance is often described with a lock-and-key analogy. There is one unique key for each lock. If you've ever had the red measles, you have antibodies (locks) against those germs (keys). You must experience red measles once, or be immunized, however, before you can develop those antibodies.

is a result of being tired. In Chapter 8, we will be discussing some allergies to drugs, but many reactions to drugs are not allergic. A host of other factors, such as an inability to break down the drug, could be the cause of symptoms.

On page 10 we describe the normal response of the immune system to harmful substances such as bacteria and viruses. But the immune system of a person with allergies reacts in a special way to some normally harmless substances that we call allergens. You might describe such an immune system as overzealous; it falsely interprets some very ordinary substances as dangerous.

Any substance that can start an allergic immune response is called an **allergen**. Allergens are generally proteins commonly found in our environment, things like particles from dust, pollen, animals and foods. They must be able to dissolve in watery secretions, and they must be small enough to penetrate the lining of the nose, lungs or digestive system.

People who are prone to allergies have a tendency to produce very large quantities of one type of antibody called **immunoglobulin E**, or IgE for short. They produce IgE in response to exposure to allergens. In allergies, as in everything else, individual responses vary greatly. A substance that causes one person to produce IgE antibodies won't bother another. Some people seem to react to only one allergen, others react to several.

How do you become sensitized?

The first time an allergic person encounters an allergen, he begins to make the specific IgE antibodies to that allergen. This is called **sensitization**. On the next encounter, that person produces more IgE antibodies, and so on. In other words, it usually takes repeated exposures to an allergen before a person has a noticeable allergic reaction.

This process of sensitization explains many confusing aspects of allergic reactions, such as why a four-year-old child suddenly reacts to a cat that has been with the family for years. It takes time and repeated exposure to an allergen to become sensitized. Some people become sensitized very quickly, while others must experience repeated exposures.

What is more puzzling is an allergic reaction that seems to occur the first time you're exposed to something, such as penicillin. You may not have realized that you were exposed to penicillin previously, but penicillin is often given to cows to treat infections in their udders. Some of it may have been transferred to milk that you drank at one time. Thus you were exposed to the drug in a hidden way.

Similarly, if a mother is breast-feeding her baby, particles from certain foods she is eating, such as peanuts and milk, may be carried through to her breast milk. If her baby is genetically susceptible to food allergies, he could become sensitized even though the only food in his diet is breast milk. Then, the first time he is given one of these other foods, he could have an allergic reaction.

The process of sensitization also explains why we can't evaluate someone for allergies until after an initial reaction. Prior to sensitization, a person does not have sufficient IgE antibodies for a positive test. Once sensitized, however, a person with allergies reacts to extremely small quantities of allergens. Throughout the entire ragweed season, a person may be exposed to just a tip of a teaspoon of pollen, and yet that would be enough to cause hay fever in a susceptible person.

In this way, allergies are very different to the reactions we call **intolerances**. A person who can eat the occasional green apple without difficulty but who feels sick after too many green apples is experiencing a form of intolerance. An allergic person, however, might have a reaction after just one bite of apple. If a person has a severe allergy, just the smell of fish or peanuts can cause a mild reaction.

A *step-by-step look at an allergic reaction*
Remember those IgE antibodies that we discussed on page 12? Once these are formed, they attach themselves to one or another of two closely related cells—either **basophil cells**, which circulate in the blood, or **mast cells**, which are concentrated in mucosal tissue.

The mucosal tissue is actually a protective layer of cells that is found in the nose and eyes. There is also mucosal tissue lining the airways, lungs, stomach and bowels. The skin, which also serves as a protective barrier, contains mast cells. Thus, it is these areas of the body that are the main trouble spots for allergic reactions.

When an allergen, such as ragweed pollen, enters your body, it stimulates certain white cells, called **macrophages** and lymphocytes, to start producing chemical messengers, the IgE antibodies. These antibodies seek out and attach themselves to either the mast cells in the mucosal tissue or the basophil cells in the blood. They then wait until the next time ragweed allergen enters the body. When it does, the IgE antibody locks onto the ragweed and holds it on the mast cell surface. The ragweed pollen is the key that unlocks a chain of chemical reactions in the mast cell.

The mast cell bursts open, releasing chemicals called **mediators** into the tissue. One of the best known mediators is **histamine**, a compound you'll be reading more about in this book. The release of mediators begins the allergic reaction and leads to **inflammation** in the tissue.

You can think of inflammation as swelling, redness and heat in an area of the body. The following are some of the ways mediators cause inflammation as part of the immediate response:

- The blood vessels expand in order to allow more blood to rush to the affected area.
- There's a "calling of the troops." That is, many specialized white cells rush to the area.
- The blood vessels leak fluid carrying the various white cells, with their chemicals and antibodies, into the affected area. The tissue swells. If the airways or nose are involved, you may notice a congested feeling. If your skin is affected, you can see the swelling.
- Mucus-producing cells in the mucosal tissue begin secreting fluids designed to trap and wash away the foreign substance. Your nose runs, your eyes weep or you cough up phlegm.
- Some muscles go into spasm. In the lungs, this could produce coughing and/or wheezing; in the bowels, it feels like cramps.

Several hours after the initial inflammation, there is a second phase of reactions, termed the **late response**, which lasts much longer. This reaction also seems to be controlled by mast cells and leads to an influx of other cells, creating further inflammation.

We are also learning that certain lymphocytes—called **T cells**—which respond to allergens, are capable of starting a cascade effect. They call in other cells and cause them to become activated, or "trigger happy," thereby creating a third mechanism for inflammation.

During this late response, inflamed tissues may over-react to changes in the weather, pollution, cigarette smoke or exercise—things that wouldn't be used in allergy skin tests but that do aggravate the patient's underlying problem.

In subsequent chapters, we will be discussing more about what happens in each organ of the body during an allergy reaction. You will be able to see how asthma, eczema and hay fever all involve inflammation in certain mucosal tissues.

Modern allergy treatment

In the past, allergy treatment focused on avoiding anything that aggravated your allergies. Now that we understand more about the inflammation process, we have medications that can regulate or turn off the inflammatory process. With these newer medications and appropriate avoidance measures, we are able to put out the sparks that ignite your disease before it becomes a raging inferno or serious attack.

By using medical treatment aggressively at this initial stage, you will be taking less medication in the long run; you will stay healthier and will not need to miss as much work or school; you won't need to be hospitalized as often for allergy reactions. These achievements weren't possible fifteen or twenty years ago, before allergists understood the late response inflammation.

Why me? Why our family?

We refer to people who make large amounts of IgE antibodies to materials such as dust, animals, pollen or foods as **atopic** individuals. This is an inherited trait. If both parents are atopic, there is a 50 to 70 per cent chance that their children will also be atopic; if one parent or sibling is atopic, the risk is 25 to 50 per cent. In addition, 10 to 15 per cent of people who have no immediate relatives with allergies become atopic.

What is actually inherited is the tendency to make excessive amounts of IgE antibodies to certain common allergens. The diseases we commonly associate with allergies—atopic dermatitis (eczema), allergic rhinitis (hay fever) and asthma—are more complicated and may be inherited separately or together. That means that if a father has hay fever, his daughter may develop asthma or hay fever or eczema, or maybe two of these conditions, or all three. The severity and pattern of illnesses varies with the individual.

By being aware of the family medical history, parents and doctors can be better prepared for certain illnesses in children. If a child is very likely to be atopic, the parents can decrease the frequency with which the child is exposed to certain allergens; the doctor can recognize the early signs of inflammation and can begin appropriate treatment sooner.

Sometimes we're fooled. A child may develop an allergy disease even before her parents show atopic patterns.

Possibly the parents had symptoms, but the disease was never diagnosed as an allergy.

The allergy diseases

In the late 1940's, the allergy diseases were defined as asthma, hay fever, eczema, migraine headaches and a few others. Allergists were doctors who specialized in treating these diseases. We now know that you can have asthma, eczema and other diseases without being atopic. The inflammation we talked about earlier can be caused in other ways. For example, asthma can be triggered by viral infections and irritants, in addition to allergies.

Allergists continue to prescribe effective treatments for non-allergic asthma, eczema and other diseases, but our approach is individualized according to the patient's problem. Thus your treatment plan may be very different from your friend's, although you may both seem to be having similar symptoms—skin rashes, itchy eyes, runny nose, difficult breathing.

Beware of alternative treatments

We expect you to think critically about what you are reading in this book. We urge you to ask your allergist or family physician questions. Do not adopt any treatment program until you are sure that your practitioner understands the true nature of allergy. Challenge the experts, and then make your own informed decisions.

Some books are almost "do-it-yourself" guides to allergy management. While we believe that patients, not doctors, manage allergies, we don't advocate taking your disease entirely into your own hands. That would be dangerous. We'll illustrate that by telling you about a young woman we've treated.

Susan occasionally had severe hives accompanied by flushing. Sometimes that would be followed by a more serious reaction involving various organs in her body. The muscles around her airways would go into spasm, making it difficult to breathe; her blood vessels would widen and there would be a sudden drop in blood pressure that would lead to unconsciousness. This condition, called anaphylaxis, may be caused by allergies.

In Susan's case, however, our tests proved that she didn't have allergies. An immune system response involves many pathways. One of the pathways in Susan would go haywire, but it wasn't allergies that would set it off—it was exercise. Therefore Susan's disease only mimicked allergy, and avoiding possible allergens certainly was of no help.

Susan's disease had a curious pattern. At certain times, usually around the time of her menstrual period, her skin became extrasensitive. If it was stroked, hives would develop. After we determined that Susan's severe reactions occurred only when her skin was extrasensitive, the treatment was straightforward. Susan was to stroke her skin daily. If she noticed a hive beginning, she was to take a very safe medication that would prevent more severe reactions from starting.

But Susan wasn't satisfied with the concept that she had an inherited biochemical problem for which there was a simple, safe treatment. She wanted to find a cause for her problems. She read extensively about food allergies, and the more she read, the more foods she began to question. She started eliminating many foods from her diet, and each time she developed hives she added new possibilities to her list of forbidden foods. But even though the list grew and grew, the restricted diet did not protect her. She became more and more panicky about identifying food allergens, instead of *concentrating on the fact that she did have a method for avoiding major reactions.*

Fortunately, Susan didn't get into great difficulty since she continued to take her medication when her skin was sensitive. However, she continued to restrict her life and her enjoyment of eating as she tried to avoid the unavoidable.

Some people are in greater jeopardy. They refuse to take medications they consider "unnatural" and instead rely on a very restricted diet and vitamin and mineral supplements, which they consider "natural." But the massive doses of nutritional supplements they are using are far too high; they can even be harmful.

We've seen so-called "natural" treatments actually harm children.

A recent case examined by the Ontario College of Physicians and Surgeons involved two children who were known to be allergic to peanut. The parents carefully avoided giving the children peanuts or any food containing peanuts.

The children also had asthma, and their mother became discouraged with the conventional management of asthma. She sought out a doctor who promised to manage the children's allergies with a diet.

Using applied kinesiology, a test with no scientific basis, the doctor decided that both children were no longer allergic to peanut. The mother then gave them pure peanut butter purchased from a health food store, but as soon as the children ate the peanut butter, they had severe allergic reactions requiring emergency treatment in a hospital.

Joey was an infant who had once had a serious allergic reaction to milk. He also tended to have mild asthma. His parents became discouraged with orthodox allergy treatment and the limitations on his diet, so they took him to a naturopath for examination. After a physical exam only, the naturopath decided that Joey had underactive adrenal and thymus glands caused by yeast infection. Proper diagnosis of these glandular problems requires certain blood tests, but the naturopath did not do these.

The naturopath prescribed thymus and adrenal extracts. One of the preparations contained milk protein and, immediately upon treatment, Joey had a severe allergic reaction. His parents had been told that he might become worse initially after treatment due to a release of toxins and therefore waited a while before taking Joey to the hospital. Fortunately, they didn't wait too long. Joey was successfully treated for the allergic reaction in a hospital emergency department.

Terry was a thirteen-year-old boy with autism. In looking for an answer to their boy's problems, the parents found an unorthodox practitioner who recommended a restricted diet. Each time Terry's autism worsened, the practitioner would eliminate more foods from his diet. But the more the diet was restricted, the worse his condition became. Finally, Terry's parents took him back to his regular doctor. He was taken off the restrictive diet and fed normal foods; he gradually improved. He had been starving.

We realize that many people become frustrated with conventional medicine and thus are attracted to some alternative therapies offered by nutritionists, herbalists or clinical ecologists. Many of these clinics sell hope—if only you will buy their products or follow their rigid regimen. But the diseases they claim to have cured are ones that often go into spontaneous remission. If the treatment doesn't work for you, they say it is because you didn't follow their instructions carefully enough.

It is often difficult for the lay person to evaluate the various clinics and treatment options. The explanations given sound just as scientific as many you hear from the established medical community. Be wary, however, if the practitioner starts talking about "subclinical deficiencies" or if he supports his theories with case histories and testimonials from former patients, rather than scientifically controlled research.

Remember, physicians and allergists can't always promise immediate results. Reliable allergy treatment often takes time. There may be no cures, but you will be able to control the symptoms.

Another danger is in becoming too complacent. People believe their disease is caused by an allergy that they've identified; they think that by avoiding the allergen, they are no longer at risk. This may simply not be true. Something else may be causing their disease and if it is left misdiagnosed or untreated, it may become more serious.

With this book, we try to help you understand the scientific basis for allergies and their safe medical treatment. Advice in this book is not meant to replace any you receive from your doctor; rather, it will make it easier for you to work with your doctor to implement both short- and long-term strategies for treating your disease.

As you read this book, you'll probably want to jump around to various chapters that discuss aspects of the diseases that are most pertinent to you. Feel free to do so, but first read Chapter 2, where we introduce some important concepts on the diagnosis of allergies. Throughout the book we've included many cross-references so that you can refer back to points you may have missed.

In Chapter 5, we suggest steps you can take to modify your environment and thus make life easier for yourself or your child. Chapter 10 is written for parents, teachers and caregivers who want to help children with these diseases enjoy life to the fullest. We hope you will pass along some of these suggestions to others who may be able to reduce allergy problems for the people they meet at school or work.

CHAPTER TWO

Diagnosing Allergies

If you or your doctor suspects you have an allergic condition, your next question will likely be, "What am I allergic to?" After all, if it's something you can avoid, you will.

But sometimes diagnosing allergies isn't as easy as we'd like it to be. We can test for a wide variety of common allergens, but first we need to have some clues as to the most likely possibilities. Each day you're exposed to dust, pollens, moulds and foods—things that cause allergy problems for some people.

To complicate matters further, sometimes allergy symptoms aren't noticeable until several hours after exposure. For example, a cat-sensitive person might not start wheezing until four to six hours after returning home from dining with friends who have a cat.

Your symptoms provide important clues, but not the complete answers. There are many other reasons, besides allergy, for a stuffy nose or an upset stomach. When you go to see an allergist, expect to answer a number of questions about your symptoms: When do they occur?

Where were you? What were you doing just before and several hours before? What was the weather like?

The following examples illustrate some of the thinking behind our questions:

- If the discharge from a runny nose is clear, allergy is a possibility; but if it is coloured, you likely have an infection.
- Mild, intermittent asthma, particularly in preschool children, often occurs without allergy, whereas chronic asthma is associated with allergy in 70 to 80 per cent of children over the age of six.
- If your eczema is very mild and patchy, it is probably not aggravated by allergies.
- Sneezing, itching and coughing around animals is often an indication of allergies in children.
- Hives or swelling immediately after drinking milk or eating foods containing egg, peanut or soy are good indications of a true food allergy.
- Sneezing or itching of the nose or eyes when outside likely indicates a pollen sensitivity. Pollen, the male reproductive cells of plants, is carried in the wind. In Ontario, tree pollen is present in April and May, grass pollen in May and June, and ragweed pollen from mid-August until the first frost. Fungal spores, reproductive cells from moulds, can cause problems from spring right through to November or December.
- We'll want to know about the medications you are taking. Even Aspirin or other ASA-containing pain relievers can cause problems. Other drugs we must consider are arthritis drugs, oral contraceptives, and beta-blocking agents for hypertension.

- Did your symptoms start soon after eating in a restaurant? That's a clue that you might be sensitive to a flavour enhancer, monosodium glutamate (MSG), or a preservative, sodium metabisulphite.

TESTING FOR ALLERGIES

Skin tests

The information we gather about your symptoms and lifestyle habits can help us decide which of the following tests are appropriate to confirm our suspicions. Usually we start with the **prick test**. This is a very simple procedure that takes only a few minutes. We place drops of solutions containing common allergen extracts on your forearm or back. Then we draw a needle through each droplet to prick the skin, so that the liquid can penetrate the surface. We don't need to go deep enough to draw blood, just enough to lift the skin surface.

Depending upon your history, there are a number of common allergens we usually test for initially, each at a different site. These are:

- Pollens. The male sex cells of plants, including trees, grasses and weeds. These are scattered by the wind and carried in the fur of animals.
- Dust and dust mites. Dust mites are very small, eight-legged creatures that you can't see with the naked eye. They feed off the dead skin cells we are constantly shedding, so they tend to be plentiful in mattresses, on upholstered furniture and in carpets. Fecal matter from the dust mite may cause allergic reactions.

- Animal dander. Dander is skin scales of animals. Usually we test with dander from cats, dogs and horses.
- Different types of moulds.
- Some foods, such as milk, egg, wheat, peanut, nuts, fish, shellfish and soy.

In one of the test sites we will use histamine, one of the mediators released during an allergic reaction. We expect this site to produce an itchy welt as an indication that your skin is responding appropriately. Because prick test results depend upon the release of histamine and other mediators from mast cells, your doctor will advise you not to take antihistamine medication before this test.

Another site will be the control site, where there is no allergen extract, just a saline (salt and water) solution. We expect no reaction here. If there is one, it is a sign your skin is overly sensitive.

After fifteen minutes, we'll examine the test sites. You may have already noticed intense itching from some sites.

A positive skin test doesn't necessarily mean you have a particular allergy. Skin test results must be considered in relation to your medical history.

A swelling and some surrounding redness at the site of the prick will indicate that you have developed IgE antibodies to that particular substance.

If the reaction is large enough, a few hours later you may notice additional swelling and heat at the site. This is from fluid and cells accumulating at the test site and is the late reaction we mentioned in the previous chapter.

When properly done, the prick test is an extremely useful way to determine if a person has an atopic immune system. It is quick, relatively inexpensive and more sensitive than blood tests. You must keep in mind, however, that skin tests show evidence of skin sensitivity only. You may not have an actual allergy problem with the substance tested. If given skin tests, up to half the population would have a localized reaction to at least one common allergen, but the number of people with allergy problems is much less. Some foods that cause a skin reaction may be eaten without difficulty. Airborne allergens, such as pollen and dust, that irritate your skin may not cause serious problems for you.

The **scratch test** is very similar to the prick test, except that first the skin is scratched and then the suspect allergen applied. It is not any more sensitive or specific than the gentler prick test, so we prefer to use the prick test instead.

The **intradermal test** involves injecting a very small amount of allergen into the skin. Although a more sensitive test, it is often less specific and is difficult to do on children, so we don't use it for routine testing. We do use it in special situations—when testing for drug sensitivities, such as an allergy to penicillin, insect stings and vaccines.

Patch tests are sometimes done by dermatologists when investigating skin rashes that they suspect are caused by various creams or ointments you are using. For this test, the substance is put on the skin and covered with a patch. One or two days later, the covering is removed and the site examined.

Skin testing may not be appropriate in some cases, such as with patients who have had certain life-threatening reactions or who have skin rashes on large areas of their bodies. In these cases, blood tests are used.

Blood tests

Many people mistakenly believe that it would be easier if the doctor took a sample of their blood and then did all the trial-and-error testing in the laboratory. But the usual blood test measures only total IgE and thus merely indicates whether you are an atopic person. This test does not tell us which substances are causing your allergy symptoms. Besides, you can have a normal total IgE and still be allergic.

We can also do a **radio-allergosorbent test (RAST)** on a sample of your blood to measure the level of IgE antibodies to specific allergens. Both these blood tests are more expensive than the skin tests, but not more sensitive. Therefore we use them only when a skin test is not appropriate.

Dietary testing

Skin testing can suggest certain food allergies, but because foods act differently when eaten than when introduced through the skin, we must resort sometimes to **challenge testing** to confirm or rule out suspected food allergies. We would never use this test if you've had a life-threatening reaction to a food, since the test involves giving you a very small amount of the food.

In **open challenge testing**, the patient knows what food is being tested. In our practice, we use this procedure with young children who, we hope, have outgrown a food allergy. By testing the child with a minute amount of food while in our offices, we can observe and, if necessary, treat any positive reactions. Our usual routine is to first touch the lip with a flake of the food and then wait twenty minutes. If there is no reaction, we then feed a small amount on the tip of a teaspoon and again wait twenty minutes. The third trial is with half a spoonful. If that is tolerated, it is safe to give a large quantity to prove that the child has outgrown the allergy.

With some symptoms, such as headaches, the power of suggestion may bring on the symptom. When we need to rule out that possibility, we can do challenge testing in a **double-blind** way. That is, neither you nor the doctor knows whether the ingredient is being ingested or not. For this kind of testing, we use a placebo, something that looks, tastes and feels the same, but has none of the suspect ingredient. Sometimes the food ingredient is freeze-dried and hidden in a gelatin capsule that you will be asked to swallow whole. The gelatin will dissolve in your stomach, releasing the test ingredient.

A good example of effective "double-blind" testing for food allergies was a research study on aspartame (Nutra-Sweet) recently done at the Duke University Medical Center. Forty people, all of whom were sure that aspartame in food caused them to have headaches, agreed to participate in the study. Dietitians served meals that did not contain aspartame, and on different days the participants swallowed gelatin capsules that either contained aspartame or no aspartame. On the test days, the aspartame dose was equivalent to four litres of diet soft drink. Each subject was asked to report all headaches and any other symptoms to a researcher who didn't know which capsule had been used that day. The number and severity of headaches was not greater, and was even a little less, on the days when the subjects had the aspartame. This double-blind study clearly proved that it wasn't the aspartame that was causing the symptoms.

In the past, **elimination diets** were often used to test for food allergies. The person was placed on a very restricted diet consisting of just a few foods—ones that rarely cause allergy symptoms, such as lamb, turkey, tuna, carrots, squash, peaches, pears, pineapple, rice and sweet potato—until all the symptoms disappeared. Then one new food was added at a time, and the person was carefully observed. This testing procedure was very tedious, required meticulous compliance and could take a long time. It could also be dangerous. Some children were kept on restricted diets that were nutritionally inadequate for long periods of time. Often their symptoms worsened due to malnutrition, but the investigators responded by restricting the diet even more.

Elimination diets were more frequently used when allergists thought it was common for a person to be allergic to many foods, but recent research has proven that very few people are allergic to more than one or two foods. Thus we believe that dietary restrictions may needlessly limit a person's lifestyle. In situations where one or a very few foods, such as milk and other dairy products, are highly suspect, we may selectively eliminate them and watch for improvement.

Unproven testing

One of our concerns is the use of testing methods that have not been validated scientifically. Although the test results are not reliable, they are used by some doctors, nutritionists, herbalists and clinical ecologists as the basis for treatment recommendations. We realize it is very difficult for patients to evaluate tests, and therefore we are going to describe some of these tests so that you can avoid them.

One such test is based on an unproven theory that foods emit a radiation to which some people are sensitive.

Testing is done without the person coming in direct contact with the food. The person is asked to hold a small bottle containing a certain food, or the vial is held near a certain organ, such as the thymus gland or ear. The patient then stretches out his arm, and the investigator feels for muscle tone. A perceived lack of muscle tone is interpreted as meaning that the person is allergic to that food. To test uncooperative small children, the child sits in the mother's lap or holds her hand, and the mother's muscle tone is then tested. This procedure is used in applied kinesiology.

Sublingual provocation and neutralization (food drops) involves placing the drops of the test material under the tongue and then observing the patient for symptoms. The treatment then consists of administering different doses of the same substance, again under the tongue, to "neutralize" and alleviate the symptoms. There is no scientific evidence that supports the effectiveness of this procedure.

With the **Vega II** or **Interro machine** the patient is attached through acupuncture needles to a computer. The machine tests for reactions without directly exposing the subject to any substance. There is no double-blind testing and no use of placebos.

Cytotoxic testing involves mixing your white blood cells with antigens. We realize it is particularly difficult for you to evaluate tests that involve sending a sample of your blood to a laboratory. But consider this: an investigator with the U.S. Food and Drug Administration sent a sample of cow's blood for mail-order cytotoxic testing. The cytotoxic laboratory did not even discover that it was cow's blood and not human blood and, for a fee of $300, sent back a report that the donor was allergic to 22 of 187 substances tested, including cow's milk, cottage cheese and yogurt.

Remember, it is your right to understand the tests and treatments your doctor is proposing. If the initial explanation doesn't make sense, ask the doctor to explain it again.

CHAPTER THREE

Asthma

There has been tremendous progress in our understanding and treatment of asthma over the past ten to fifteen years. With modern treatment, patients with asthma can now look forward to a better quality of life.

UNDERSTANDING ASTHMA

Medical research has significantly advanced our understanding and treatment of asthma. At the same time, however, there is a world-wide increase in the frequency of severe illness and death from the disease. The reasons for this increase are not completely understood. Whatever the cause, doctors believe that if these asthmatics had had the benefit of proper diagnosis and had been treated earlier in the course of the disease, many would have lived.

Wheezing and coughing
The hallmark of asthma is wheezing, with difficulties in breathing caused by a narrowing of the airways to the

> **How the lungs work**
>
> All the cells in your body need a constant supply of oxygen. The role of your lungs is to bring that supply of oxygen into your body, to transfer the oxygen to the blood and to remove the waste gas (carbon dioxide) from the blood and your body. To do this, the two lobes of lung in your chest cavity have a very efficient design that results in an inner surface area equivalent to a full-sized tennis court. Inside the lungs are millions of tiny air sacs, called alveoli, connected to a series of branching pipes— the bronchial tubes. The alveoli and bronchial tubes resemble bunches of grapes attached to a vine. The air that you breathe in travels down your windpipe, through the bronchial tubes to the alveoli. There the oxygen is transferred to the blood stream, and carbon dioxide is removed from the blood.
>
> Lining the bronchial tubes is mucosal tissue, the type of tissue we discussed in Chapter 1 as being important during allergy reactions (see page 14).

lungs. But not all people with asthma wheeze. In some asthmatics, the only symptom is coughing, most often at night and first thing in the morning or with exertion. The coughing happens practically every day and is persistent. Others notice only shortness of breath when climbing stairs or exercising. Because both patients and doctors don't pay enough attention to these symptoms, the diagnosis of asthma is often missed. Other times, the disease is misdiagnosed as bronchitis, a persistent viral infection or even recurrent pneumonia.

What goes wrong in asthma?

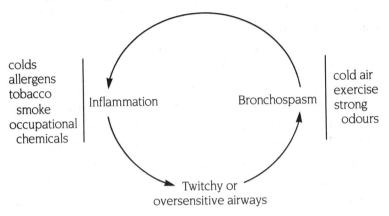

On page 36, we've described how healthy lungs work. In a person with asthma, several changes occur in the bronchial tubes as illustrated above. The mucosal lining becomes inflamed—it swells, thus narrowing the airway, and excess mucus or phlegm is produced. The mucus can form a sticky plug that further narrows the bronchial passages. The primary causes of such inflammation are viral infections (such as colds), allergens (including pollens, dust, animal dander and moulds), occupational chemicals (fumes in paint and plastic factories) and tobacco smoke.

As part of the inflammation process, many different cells invade the mucosal lining. These cells contain chemical substances that are released and lead to a twitchiness or oversensitivity of the bronchial tubes. Once the airways become inflamed and overly sensitive, they respond more easily to certain triggers such as cold air, exercise and irritating odours.

The end result of this cascade of events is the production of asthmatic symptoms, one of which is a tightening of the bronchial muscles, or **bronchospasm**, which further narrows the airways. Thus, airway inflammation is the basic problem and bronchospasm is an end result. If allowed to continue, the symptoms are aggravated.

In the past, we defined asthma as reversible airway obstruction and we concentrated on opening the airways with bronchodilators, medications that relax the muscles lining the bronchial passages. Now, however, we recognize that the source of the problem is the inflammation of the lining of the bronchial passages caused by a variety of factors, some known and some unknown. Whatever the cause, our treatment is aimed at reducing the inflammation.

Airway inflammation may lead to persistent coughing, wheezing and shortness of breath—the triad of symptoms associated with asthma. Coughing is a reflex action of the chest and diaphragm muscles trying to force air quickly out through the bronchi to dislodge mucus plugs. Wheezing is a whistle-like sound that results from blowing air through a narrowed tube. Patients may also notice a feeling of chest tightness, gasping and difficulty in breathing, as well as a generalized feeling of apprehension.

Although the above symptoms may be intermittent, the inflammation of the mucosal tissue continues much longer. Between attacks, an asthma sufferer may feel comfortable, but his inflamed lungs could be operating at much below peak capacity.

ASTHMA IN CHILDREN

In our practice, we treat many children with asthma. It is a very complex disease in which allergies can play a part, but to blame all asthma on allergies and treat it as such would be far too simplistic. As a matter of fact, viral infections (colds) are a far more common trigger of asthma in young children.

In the past, we would rarely diagnose asthma in children under the age of three. Only patients who had wheezing were considered asthmatic. Those who had recurrent or persistent cough and/or rattly chests were thought to have bronchitis or chronic viral infections. We now recognize that the majority of such patients have asthma with attacks triggered by viral infections.

Any child with persistent or recurrent coughing, or coughing with chest congestion following a cold, should be evaluated for asthma. The hallmark features are a cough that worsens at night or in the early morning, or with exposure to cold air or various odours, or following exercise.

Recently we conducted a survey among 1,500 children under the age of five in two urban communities, Mississauga and Brampton, Ontario. Approximately 10 per cent of the children had had a session of wheezing in the previous year and another 8 to 9 per cent had had coughing. That is, almost one in five of the children had chestiness, a statistic that is similar to that in other countries.

At the age of three, Martin was brought to us because, with each cold, he was coughing a lot. His doctor had diagnosed his problem as croup or bronchitis and had treated him with antibiotics and cough syrup. But it wasn't helping.

When we questioned his mother, we found that Martin coughed most mornings upon waking up, or whenever he became excited. Even though the coughing worsened with a cold, he was not in grave danger. But his coughing was keeping the family up at night.

Martin's history didn't indicate any signs of allergy. He had tolerated milk, wheat, eggs and peanut butter when they were introduced into his diet. He had no symptoms around animals. With colds he did have a runny nose, but the discharge was primarily green, not clear, as it would be if he had hay fever. Between colds he had no runny nose or sneezing. Nevertheless, we tested him for allergies using the prick test method and confirmed that he was non-allergic.

On close questioning, we found that Martin had a history of coughing with colds since about eighteen months of age. Then the coughing would last about two weeks. Once he entered day care, the frequency of colds was greater. During the winter, he never seemed to be free of symptoms. Thus Martin is typical of a young child who has asthma caused by viral infections, not allergies.

Although there are other causes for chronic wheezing in a young child (see page 41), asthma is the most common reason. Martin is typical in that he never actually wheezed, or perhaps his parents did not recognize a wheeze and instead identified the problem as a "rattling" noise in his chest. It is believed that 15 per cent of young children develop asthma.

The main causes of childhood asthma are viral respiratory tract infections, allergy and second-hand cigarette smoke. We also believe that other factors, such as environmental pollutants, cold air, strong odours and exercise can irritate already inflamed airways and bring on an attack of wheezing and coughing.

Colds and childhood asthma

It is completely normal for younger children to have frequent head colds. After all, it's virtually impossible to

Other causes of wheezing in children

Although asthma is by far the most common cause of persistent and/or recurrent coughing and wheezing in childhood, there are other rarer causes, which your doctor should consider. In infants under a year of age, especially in winter and early spring, we often see viral infections in which wheezing is a main feature. This is usually bronchiolitis, and it isn't until a child has had two such episodes that we consider asthma as a possibility. Even the first episode of wheezing after a cold, however, can signal the beginning of asthma.

Preschool children often swallow objects, even undigested food, which can be inhaled into the lungs. Routine chest x-rays or more specialized x-rays can rule out this possibility.

Cystic fibrosis is a rare, inherited disease, affecting one in 1,600 to 2,000 children. That's much more infrequent than the one in five who have asthma. This disease causes abnormalities in the lungs and in the digestion of food. The children fail to gain weight, have abnormal bowel movements and may have multiple chest infections with wheezing. We diagnose this disease with a test that measures the amount of salt in a child's perspiration.

There are other rare causes of wheezing, including structural abnormalities since birth. Again, routine and special x-rays can rule out these problems.

protect children from exposure to viral infections, the cause of the common cold. Young children attending day care or school have a good chance of picking up a viral infection every few weeks. Children are likely to have a blocked nose, laboured breathing and a cough for a few days when they have a cold.

> **Signs of asthma**
> - **prolonged cough or chestiness with colds**
> - **frequent colds, every two to three weeks**
> - **recurrent croup**
> - **shortness of breath after exercise**
> - **recurrent pneumonia**

However, we believe that if a child is chesty with each cold and if the chestiness lasts two to three weeks with each cold, she should be investigated and treated for asthma, as viral infections can create enormous inflammation in the airways. We also suspect asthma if she has recurrent croup, or a prolonged cough, or recurrent shortness of breath after exercise or recurrent pneumonia. Recurrent is the key word. With all the viruses around, single episodes of chestiness are normal. But when such illnesses are repeated, it's time to consider management with asthma medication. Otherwise, the next infection could trigger a serious attack requiring emergency hospital treatment.

At one point in the past, Martin had been treated with medication designed to relax the muscles around the bronchial tubes and stop muscle spasm. Such medication is classified as a bronchodilator. Although it usually provides immediate relief, it is essentially a "quick-fix" approach, as it doesn't treat the underlying inflammation.

We treated Martin more aggressively with medication designed to reduce the inflammation in his airways (an anti-inflammatory medication). After three weeks, medication was discontinued as Martin was no longer coughing. With subsequent colds, medication was restarted early and the chestiness cleared quickly. Martin will continue to need medication intermittently until he "outgrows" his asthma.

Anti-inflammatory medications are useful with infants who are not allergic but who tend to wheeze or become chesty with each cold. Sometimes children develop a persistent "100-day" cough following whooping cough or a similar illness. Then, asthma medication helps recovery and these children have a good chance of outgrowing the problem. While anti-inflammatory medications cannot cure asthma, they can reduce the severity of symptoms.

Allergies and asthma

There is a group of children who may or may not have had chestiness with viral infections as preschoolers, but who, as they get older, develop symptoms suggestive of allergies—sneezing, running nose, itching or rubbing of eyes and nose. Some of these children may also have asthma symptoms that are triggered by allergens such as pollens, animal dander, dust mites or moulds. In fact, for about 60 to 80 per cent of asthmatic children over the age of six, the disease is associated with allergies.

Andrew was brought to us when he was almost seven years old. His doctor had diagnosed asthma a year earlier and had been treating Andrew with a bronchodilator. But his mother was concerned that Andrew wasn't doing as well as he should. He lacked energy and wasn't able to participate fully in sports because he would start wheezing, which would continue even after he'd stopped exercising. On cold winter days, he would also have breathing problems when walking to school.

Once, when he had a cold, he coughed so hard he had to be treated at the hospital. Since starting to use the bronchodilator, however, he hadn't required further emergency hospital treatment, but he still wasn't as healthy as he should be.

When we questioned his parents about his medical history, we found that he'd had mild, patchy eczema when very young. He hadn't had any problems associated with foods, but his mother had noticed some problems when he was around cats, although the family had no pets at home.

Sometimes he had an itchy nose and would sneeze, suggesting nasal allergy. On physical examination, we did find stuffiness in the nose and the lining of the nose was swollen. The family hadn't noticed any seasonal variations, except for the fact that his wheezing became worse with winter colds. Since about age two, Andrew had had chestiness with colds. His cough would last ten to fourteen days, and he was often treated with antibiotics. Instead of improving as he got older, he actually got worse.

On the basis of Andrew's medical history and the physical examination, we suspected he had allergies. Skin tests confirmed our suspicions; Andrew did test positive to cat dander, dust mites and ragweed. It is likely that his allergies are responsible for the worsening of his asthma symptoms over the previous year. His asthma was of a mild, but chronic, nature.

Although using the bronchodilator had provided symptomatic relief, it did not reduce the inflammation. This meant that any time Andrew developed a cold, the inflammation caused by the virus, on top of inflammation of allergy, would worsen his symptoms.

We treated Andrew with an anti-inflammatory medication to bring his asthma under control. We also taught his parents about measures for environmental control, especially with regard to dust and cat exposure. We warned them to watch him closely during ragweed season, that is, midsummer to mid-fall. There was a good chance his asthma might worsen then.

September is a particularly busy time in our offices. Children are returning to classrooms, where they will be exposed to viral infections right in the midst of the pollen season. Thus, they are exposed to a double whammy—two common causes of asthma.

Many children over the age of three, like Andrew, are allergic to cat dander. This isn't cat hair, but dead skin cells. During the winter, when the cat enjoys staying inside, the dander accumulates throughout the house. To the parents and family doctor it may seem that the child has frequent colds, which are managed with cough syrup and antibiotics. No one recognizes the child's sensitivity to the family cat because the symptoms tend to be constant. The cat doesn't need to enter the room to trigger an asthma response. Its dander is already there. Dander from dogs and other animals, and even birds, also causes allergies, although not as frequently.

Families love their pets, and find it extremely hard to give up a cat or dog. If they don't, they must recognize the choice they're making.

But animal dander isn't the only allergen associated with asthma. Dust, pollens and moulds can trigger asthma in some children. We look for allergies in every asthmatic child and, if there are any, we tell the parents that it is worth taking steps to avoid the allergen, as it can mean that less medication may be necessary. In children born to allergic parents, it is even more important to start early preventive measures to avoid allergy sensitization. These include avoidance measures such as dust control and ensuring animal-free homes. Further steps for avoidance of allergens are given in Chapter 5.

> **Over and over again, it's been proven that second-hand cigarette smoke increases chestiness in children.**

Sometimes avoidance just isn't possible. Children with very severe asthma are often sensitive to many things in their environment, and to try to avoid all allergens would mean that they would have to be isolated from normal life. Because of the modern asthma medications discussed later in this chapter, such extreme measures are not necessary.

There is one irritant, however, that we believe families should make a conscientious effort to eliminate—cigarette smoke, both in the home and in the car. In a study we did of 600 children with asthma seen at The Hospital for Sick Children in Toronto, we found that one-third were living in homes where there was a smoker. Some families spend considerable money on renovations to their home to reduce some allergens but continue to expose their children to second-hand cigarette smoke.

Asthma in older children and adolescents
In early childhood, asthma is twice as common in boys as it is in girls. During adolescence, these male-to-female ratios tend to equalize. In the younger group, asthma attacks are usually triggered by viral infection, whereas children who develop asthma when they are older

are more likely to have their asthma associated with allergies.

We do know that teenagers tend to rebel against the restrictions of any chronic disease, including asthma. They are less compliant when it comes to monitoring their lung capacity and taking medications. Generally, they prefer to rely on bronchodilators—the "quick fixes"—rather than take the anti-inflammatory medications. All too often they allow their asthma to deteriorate significantly before seeking medical help.

Yet the best treatment for adolescents is the same as for children and adults—aggressive reduction of the inflammation in the airways and avoidance, where possible, of allergens or irritants that they know are likely to trigger an attack.

ASTHMA IN ADULTS

Asthma may be diagnosed for the first time during the adult years, although the person may have had, as a child, asthma that went undiagnosed. In some cases, the delayed onset of asthma may be due to first-time exposure to chemicals or fumes at work.

All too often the coughing and sputum production of asthma in adults is blamed on smoking; shortness of breath and fatigue with exercise may be felt to be due to poor physical conditioning. However, any person who experiences repeated episodes of coughing, shortness of breath or wheezing—especially at night, after exercise or on exposure to cold air or irritating fumes—should be evaluated for the possibility of asthma. Do not wait until you end up in an emergency department with breathing difficulties.

Unfortunately, the diagnosis of asthma may at times be difficult. A physical examination, blood tests and a chest x-ray may help in the diagnosis, but in some people the results are normal even though the person does have asthma. Even breathing tests may appear normal. The clues that you do have a problem should be in your answers to the doctor's questions: Do you regularly cough at night or in the morning? Do you experience shortness of breath when exercising or climbing stairs? Do your symptoms worsen during the spring, summer or fall? Are your symptoms better on weekends or when you are on vacation? Do you notice your symptoms change when the barometric pressure changes? Are you taking Aspirin or medications for arthritis (see page 51)? Do you or any members of your family smoke? Are there smokers near you at work? Have you had difficulty breathing after eating certain foods or after eating in certain restaurants?

If the answers to some of these questions are "yes," the doctor may suggest a trial with anti-asthma medications even if the results of the tests listed previously are normal.

Asthma during pregnancy

The hormonal and physical changes in your body during pregnancy may worsen your asthma—or make it better. About one-third of pregnant women with asthma find their condition improves, one-third say it worsens, and the rest don't notice any change. If you do experience greater difficulty in breathing, it will likely be during the last trimester, when your growing baby is occupying ever-increasing space in your abdomen.

As a general rule, medications of any kind are discouraged during pregnancy, unless absolutely necessary. That also applies to medications you use to control your asthma. Asthma medications, however, are often essential. Without treatment, the tissues in the mother's lungs become swollen and unable to function properly. She will have difficulty breathing and sleeping. The supply of oxygen in her blood will decrease. Since all the oxygen for a developing fetus comes through the mother's blood supply, the oxygen supply to her fetus could also be compromised. If the mother's asthma is poorly controlled, the fetus could have problems developing normally. Statistics show that uncontrolled asthma in the mother increases the risk of prematurity, low birth weight and complications at the time of delivery.

With your doctor's guidance, you should be able to manage your asthma for optimal breathing and comfort. Your goal will be full control, with no wheezing, no night or early morning cough and no shortness of breath. When it is time for delivery, you'll need to be able to breathe deeply.

Your doctor may need to adjust your medications during pregnancy and will advise you to avoid certain ones close to your due date, as these could interfere with normal labour.

By avoiding allergens and irritants, you may be able to reduce your dependence on medications. During your pregnancy, be forceful in insisting that your friends not smoke in your presence or in your home or car. Think about the other things that irritate your lungs and take steps to eliminate them, as much as possible, from your life. There is absolutely no evidence that asthma or allergies in the mother increase the risk of congenital defects or malformations.

Asthma in the elderly

The older generation is probably the group most over-looked when it comes to asthma treatment. Rather than wheezing, symptoms in the elderly tend to be shortness of breath, coughing and sputum production. These are often mistaken for signs of chronic bronchitis or heart disease. It's also possible for asthma to coexist with bronchitis—in which case, both should be aggressively treated.

Even if the right diagnosis is made, elderly asthma patients may do poorly for a number of reasons. Some forget to take their medications; some lack the coordination necessary to use their inhalers; others have an increased tendency to experience side effects from the medication. As with all patients, it is particularly important to monitor the progress of the elderly and adjust the treatment to the individual's state of health and special needs.

Occupational asthma

In approximately 5 per cent of adult asthmatics, chemicals encountered at work create or worsen their condition. (The two most common chemicals that cause asthma are TDI, toluene diisocyanate, widely used in the electronic and foam industries, and TMA, trimetallic anhydride, a widely used epoxy resin.) Consider this possibility if your asthma improves during vacations, or if wheezing, coughing or chest congestion frequently starts while you are at work. These symptoms could also start in the evening, several hours after you leave work.

Occupational asthma is still a possibility even if you've been working for several years in the same plant without difficulty. After all, it takes months and even years to become sensitized.

Conditions that may worsen asthma

A number of conditions may complicate or worsen asthma—infections in the lungs, chronic lung disease from smoking, heart problems or any reflux of stomach acids upwards into the esophagus. Some women find that asthma worsens at certain times during their menstrual cycle.

Medications containing acetylsalicylic acid (ASA), such as Aspirin and many arthritis medications, can also aggravate asthma. Beta-blocking drugs, used to treat heart problems, high blood pressure and glaucoma, may unmask underlying asthma conditions or worsen them. In fact, most allergists won't do complicated testing or start some treatments while a patient is on a beta-blocker. Thus, every doctor who is treating you should know that you have asthma so that alternative medications may be used.

Emotional stresses can worsen symptoms of asthma but not cause it. Conversely, asthma contributes to personal stress, especially if it is not well controlled. It's not unexpected that someone who must worry about exposure to cold, smoke, dust or pollens, or who must take medication several times a day, would become anxious. But the aggressive treatment we will be discussing later, along with a better understanding of asthma, can help in reducing your concerns about the disease. The more you gain confidence that you can do something to control your asthma, the better you'll feel.

DIAGNOSING ASTHMA

In addition to taking a detailed history and doing a physical examination, allergists can use a few specialized diagnostic tools, if your symptoms warrant them. Chest x-rays may be taken to rule out other causes of wheezing and breathing difficulties, but a chest x-ray cannot show asthma.

The **pulmonary function test** consists of blowing into a special machine that calculates the rate of airflow through your lungs. If there is inflammation in your lungs, the flow rate will be significantly reduced.

Another test, the **histamine** or **methacholine challenge**, measures whether the airflow through your lungs is reduced after inhaling these chemicals. This helps us to determine the sensitivity or twitchiness of your airways. Normal test results, however, do not rule out the possibility of asthma. Also, in the very young or the elderly it is not always feasible to do these tests. Therefore, when the tests are normal but asthma is still strongly suspected, a trial with anti-asthma medications is warranted to see if your symptoms improve.

MANAGEMENT OF ASTHMA

By now you've probably realized that we treat asthma very aggressively. We want to do more than simply relieve the person's current symptoms—coughing, wheezing, shortness of breath and chest tightness; we want to reduce the underlying inflammation that causes the swelling and mucus production, so that flare-ups of the asthma are not as frequent, nor as severe.

Often symptoms can be so mild the person doesn't realize that the coughing, wheezing or shortness of breath are signs of asthma. But these symptoms should serve as an early warning that there is inflammation in the bronchial tubes that requires treatment.

We want to help our patients to be free of the triad of asthma symptoms—coughing, wheezing and shortness of breath—at night, in the morning and with exercise. When that goal is successfully reached, the person with asthma is definitely happier and healthier.

> **With effective asthma management, patients should be able to live completely normal lives—working, studying and playing as much as they want, without worrying about coughing, wheezing or shortness of breath.**

This should be achieved with as few daily medications as possible and with no harmful side effects. It can be achieved in the majority of patients with mild or moderate asthma. They will need medications at times, but often not on a regular basis. Others, with more severe asthma, will require ongoing medications to achieve this optimal control. A very few asthmatics who have a severe form of the disease will continue to have some symptoms. For these patients, the best treatment is regular medication with a minimum of side effects.

During your first visits, the doctor will explain the nature of your disease and the relevance of possible trigger factors. The presence or absence of allergy should be established in order to recommend avoidance strategies that will be useful for you. The doctor will then recommend management goals, both short- and long-term;

establish a time frame for achieving these goals; and discuss the types of medications that can help you to reach these goals. You'll also need to know about possible side effects from the medications and when to call your doctor if these occur. Since many of the medications are inhaled, the doctor will also teach you how to use an inhaling device that sprays the medication directly into your airways.

Ultimately you (or the parents, in the case of a young child) are responsible for managing your own asthma. Therefore, you must understand the nature of inflammation in asthma, how medication deals with inflammation and how to use the medication properly.

In the past, asthma management generally involved using bronchodilators (drugs that relieve the spasm in the muscles lining the bronchial tubes), allergy shots (to control the allergies triggering the asthma attacks) and environmental controls (measures to remove or reduce the many allergens and irritants in the patient's home).

Today there is much greater emphasis on reducing the inflammation in the airways. We use bronchodilators less frequently and we rarely give allergy shots. Environmental control is still important, but it is no longer necessary to place undue restrictions on your life. Modern asthma management involves achieving a reasonable balance between environmental controls and medications.

Environmental control
We believe that environmental control is helpful and therefore we've written an entire chapter (Chapter 5) on practical steps you can take to reduce the level of dust, moulds, animal dander, pollens and irritating odours in your home and at work or school. Tobacco smoke and

animal dander are usually the worst offenders but we will also discuss ways to reduce your exposure to other factors, as well.

At first, you may not see the link between your environment and your symptoms, and you may hesitate to follow some of these suggestions. You should realize, however, that whenever there is inflammation in your airways, you are more sensitive. Then, things such as cold air or strong odours that don't normally bother you may aggravate your asthma. Therefore it makes sense to learn about and avoid, when possible, things that are likely to initiate or aggravate your asthma.

Allergy shots

At one time, many people with asthma were routinely given allergy shots. The hope was that by gradually exposing the person to increasing doses of the common allergens, he would build up a level of tolerance. In fact, allergy shots are only marginally useful and are appropriate only for those people whose asthma is caused by a clearly defined allergen, such as ragweed. Today, if allergy shots are used, they should be as an adjunct to anti-inflammatory treatments and should be continued only if there is a definite, measurable improvement.

ASTHMA MEDICATIONS

There are two main groups of asthma medications—the anti-inflammatory medications and the bronchodilators—and there are two forms in which they are normally taken—as swallowed medications or as inhaled medications. We usually refer to the former as oral drugs; they may be either tablets or liquid. In most instances, we recommend the inhaled medications as they go straight to the target organ and thus can be used in lower doses than the oral medications.

Anti-inflammatory medications

These medications reduce inflammation in the lining of the airways. We generally use sodium cromoglycate (Intal), nedocromil sodium (Tilade), ketotifen (Zaditen) or the more powerful inhaled steroids.

Non-steroid medications. With children, we may start with Intal as it is very safe and effective with mild asthma. When the drug originally became available, over 20 years ago, it was thought to control the development of asthma symptoms by blocking the release of mediators from the mast cells. We now believe it controls inflammation in other ways. During an asthma attack, Intal should be used along with a bronchodilator medication.

Tilade is a newer anti-inflammatory which is slightly more powerful than Intal. Both Tilade and Intal are available in puffer form, with two puffs of the inhaler, four times a day, being the usual dose for children. Intal can also be given by nebulizer solution.

Zaditen is an oral medication, available in either liquid or pill form, with both antihistamine and anti-asthma properties. It is not very powerful but can be used very easily in children under three years who have mild asthma but fight the use of inhaled medication.

All these medications have very few side effects which are relatively minor. The appropriate choice of medication should be discussed with your doctor.

Steroid medications. These are the most effective anti-inflammatory agents currently available. With steroids, we are able to decrease the "hectic" pace of recurrent or persistent coughing and wheezing. For some asthmatics, a short course of oral steroids has resulted in less medication use overall.

> **A short course of steroids can provide dramatic relief from symptoms and greatly improve overall asthma treatment.**

We should point out that the steroids we use in the treatment of asthma are not the same ones that have been used illegally by athletes. Those are "anabolic" steroids. For asthma, we prescribe "corticosteroids."

In Canada, we can choose from a number of inhaled steroids (Beclovent, Vanceril, Becloforte, Pulmicort, Flovent, Bronalide and Azmacort). Common side effects—hoarse throat and fungal infection (thrush) in the mouth and throat—can be reduced by rinsing your mouth and throat after each treatment or using a spacer device attached to your inhaler. A major concern is that patients on very high doses (400 micrograms or more) could suffer from impaired growth. The newer drugs, Pulmicort and Flovent, are less likely to cause this problem than the older agents. While inhaled steroids are safer than oral steroid, the need for high doses indicates a high level of asthma and your doctor should monitor you carefully.

When the inhaled steroids aren't effective enough, it may be necessary to use an oral steroid, prednisone, for a short period of time—one to two weeks. Such short bursts of use are not associated with side effects, but prolonged daily use is generally avoided as the possible side effects are many—weight gain, puffy face, swollen feet, fatigue, muscle weakness and cramps, mood changes, sleep disturbances, increased appetite, nausea, vomiting, diarrhea, bone pain, hip damage, cataracts, bruises, acne, sugar in the urine and increased blood pressure. If taken for a long period of time, prednisone may impair bone growth or delay sexual maturation in children. This is certainly not a drug to be used indiscriminately; close monitoring, by the doctor, of the dosage and any problems is essential.

Our list of side effects and precautions may seem frightening, but please realize that your doctor carefully considers both risks and benefits. When started soon enough and used at the appropriate dose for a reasonable period of time, steroids can greatly improve the course of asthma without significant problems with side effects. If patients resist treatment, their asthma can quickly worsen. They may be hospitalized and risk death. Steroids have saved lives.

Bronchodilators

The **beta agonists** (Ventolin, Alupent, Berotec, Bricanyl, Pro-Air, Serevent) open the airways by relaxing the muscles that encircle the bronchial tubes. They can provide dramatic relief from wheezing, coughing or difficult breathing, and therefore we call them the "quick fixes."

In the past, the bronchodilators were used as first-line treatment. Patients were taught to use these medications whenever they experienced breathing problems. We now believe you should fight asthma as you would a fire, when it is just a few sparks, before it becomes

> **If you are using a bronchodilator more than twice a week and the symptoms persist, this is a sign the inflammation is getting worse. It is time for aggressive treatment—anti-inflammatory medication.**

a raging inferno. The first "sparks" are usually night or morning cough; wheezing is the "inferno." That means we aggressively treat any inflammation with the anti-inflammatory drugs until the patient is completely stabilized. Then we will reduce the medication gradually, watching for any return of symptoms.

There will still be times when using a bronchodilator is necessary—during a viral infection, when there is a flare-up of your symptoms in the ragweed season or if you have difficulty breathing after exercise. A bronchodilator may also be used along with an anti-inflammatory medication during an asthma attack. Then the usual dose is one to two puffs, two to four times a day. Frequent or daily use of bronchodilators alone is no longer warranted. It indicates that the patient needs an anti-inflammatory medication.

There are also side effects associated with the use of bronchodilators—tremors, shakiness, rapid heartbeat, restlessness, inability to sleep or headaches. These may disappear with a lowered dose or with more controlled use.

Theophylline drugs also relieve bronchospasm, but in a different way than beta agonist bronchodilators. These oral medications (Choledyl, Quibron, Elixophyllin, Theolair, Theo-Dur and Somophyllin-12) were used more commonly in the past, before the safer, inhaled anti-inflammatory medications became available. The side effects with the theophylline drugs are numerous and can include hyperactivity, sleep disturbances, poor attention span and behaviour problems—as well as numerous digestive problems. These drugs can even cause vomiting of blood and seizures.

Atropine-like medications (Atrovent) also help relieve bronchospasm, but by a different mechanism again.

These medications can be effective in the initial treatment of severe asthma attacks and can provide an additive effect when used in combination with conventional bronchodilating drugs, such as Ventolin.

Serevent is a new bronchodilator which remains active for 12 hours. It can't provide immediate relief but it is useful in patients who are taking high doses of inhaled steroid daily, yet still experiencing breakthrough symptoms.

Other drugs used by asthmatics

Contrary to previous thinking, **antihistamines** do not dry mucus secretions in the lungs and therefore can be used by people with asthma to relieve nasal symptoms. Zaditen has both antihistamine properties and anti-asthma properties. It can be useful in mild childhood asthma.

Antibiotics are occasionally prescribed if there is a bacterial infection. Antibiotics are ineffective in treating viral infections, such as the common cold, and they do not cure asthma. Generally, asthma medications are more appropriate than antibiotics when your child has asthma aggravated by a cold.

The same applies to **cough medicines**. Asthmatics who cough will benefit more from the appropriate dose of their asthma medication than from a cough medicine.

Inhaling devices

Inhaled medications go directly into the airways and thus can achieve the same effect with a lower dose than would be necessary with an oral medication. However, to get the most benefit from the medication, you must understand how to use the inhaler properly.

There are a number of inhaling devices available, as well as extension tubes and compressors. No one is ideal;

some trials may be necessary to find the ones that work best for you. With children, their needs may change as they grow.

Puffers, or metered-dose inhalers, are a convenient way for children to carry and use their medications. As we will discuss in Chapter 10, as soon as a child demonstrates responsibility, she should be allowed to keep her puffer with her so it is readily available as soon as needed. Overuse of a puffer does not indicate addiction, rather it is a sign that the asthma is not under control.

In stressful situations even children who have learned to use a puffer may not do it properly. For this reason, the doctor should regularly review the technique.

Aerochambers are tube-like devices into which various inhalers can be inserted. With them, you spray first and then inhale, making it easier to use by young children or patients who lack coordination. They are also helpful in reducing the mouth and throat side effects from inhaled steroids. Some aerochambers have a face mask attached, others have a mouthpiece.

Powdered inhalers are also helpful for patients who lack coordination, as the medicine is inhaled only when a breath is taken. These devices allow you to measure the amount of drug more accurately. The choice of the inhaler depends upon the drug you are using. The Rotahaler and Diskhaler can deliver Ventolin or Beclovent; the Spinhaler is used for Intal; and the Turbuhaler delivers Bricanyl and Pulmicort. These dry powder delivery systems are being improved and may one day replace the puffers.

Compressors are electrical or battery-driven motorized devices that deliver a fine mist through a mask. They can be used for drugs such as Ventolin, Atrovent and Intal and may be used for steroid preparations.

Normal breathing for approximately ten minutes is all that is required to inhale all the medication. Compressors are especially useful with young children who cannot use the aerochamber devices effectively. Staff from the hospital or equipment supplier can teach you how to use and maintain these devices.

THE ASTHMA ACTION PLAN

The action plan is a tool by which the patient can control his asthma, instead of allowing the disease to run his life. The doctor and patient establish certain individualized guidelines as to when to start medications, the type and dosage, when the frequency and amount of medication needs to be changed, when and what other medications should be added and at what point the patient should call the doctor or seek immediate additional medical help. A well-understood action plan reduces apprehension, especially at times when the physician is unavailable.

One method you may use to gauge your progress, while following the action plan, is the peak flow meter. This provides a number that represents the amount of air that can be expelled from the lungs as fast as possible. The flow rate, measured in litres per minute, correlates to some degree with the amount of obstruction in the lungs. To use the peak flow meter, you take as deep a breath as you can, then blow into the meter. The best of three such blows is recorded. It is ideally done in the morning and at night. Although it may be difficult to complete peak flow meter readings daily, they certainly should be taken anytime you are ill or changing medications. Once a patient knows his normal peak flow value, keeping the value within 10 per cent should be the goal. The way a patient feels cannot always serve as an accurate barometer of what is occurring inside the lungs. The peak flow measure provides a more accurate assessment.

A successful action plan for asthma management involves three steps:

- bringing your asthma under control;
- maintaining asthma control;
- stepping up treatment when asthma starts to get out of control.

Bringing your asthma under control. Initial treatment is designed to aggressively attack the disease and bring it under control. Full control means no coughing, wheezing or shortness of breath at night, in the morning, with exercise or after exposure to cold air or various irritants.

If you have only mild symptoms for a few days at a time, we may start with one of the bronchodilating medications delivered through an appropriate inhaling device. We would expect your symptoms to be fully cleared and the medication use stopped within five or six days. Inhaler use should not exceed four times a day. If that isn't achievable, it is an indication that inflammation is already present in the walls of the bronchial tubes. You will need one of the anti-inflammatory medications—Intal or an inhaled steroid. If the asthma is still not controlled, we would increase the inhaled steroid dose or, if necessary, add an oral steroid.

In severe cases, we will start with either inhaled or oral steroids, or both. We must be careful not to underestimate the initial level of asthma, as the disease could worsen during the time the aggressive treatment is delayed.

Maintaining asthma control. Once you are stable and symptom-free, the medication will be gradually reduced to the lowest level necessary to keep you symptom-free. Some patients may need to continue with a maintenance dose of anti-inflammatory medication, while others will need no routine medications.

Stepping up treatment when asthma starts to get out of control. Any time there is a return of symptoms or a fall in the peak flow measurements by more than 10 per cent, the anti-inflammatory agent is immediately re-introduced, or the frequency or dosage increased, until full control is again achieved. A bronchodilator may also be needed to provide quick symptom relief. If a patient needs to use a bronchodilator on a regular basis, we know that full control has not been achieved.

With a few patients who have very severe asthma, we must balance the goal of full control with the need to keep the dose of medications at a safe level.

Examples of asthma treatment

The following cases illustrate the complexity of asthma and asthma treatments.

> *Helena was eight years old when she came to our offices for treatment of her asthma. As a younger child, she'd had just two episodes of wheezing—each time with a cold that lasted ten to fourteen days. About a year ago, she again had a viral infection with a runny nose, coughing and then wheezing. Her parents took her to the emergency department of the hospital, where she was given a bronchodilator to use intermittently whenever she had difficulty breathing. By the time we saw her, she was needing the bronchodilator at least twice a week. She would cough most mornings and nights*

and was often short of breath following exercise. These are symptoms of unstable asthma.

One day, when Helena was holding her cat, she suddenly began coughing and wheezing severely. She was having so much difficulty breathing that she became hysterically frightened. Her mother noticed that she was turning blue. Helena was experiencing a severe asthma attack. She had good reason to be hysterical—she could barely breathe. The airways to and from her lungs were blocked.

Helena's mother immediately gave her the bronchodilator to open up the tubes to her lungs. Although Helena's response was slow, her sudden attack did end. The bronchodilator had provided the necessary quick fix.

We conducted allergy tests that confirmed that Helena was allergic to cat dander, but to no other common allergens. The family gave up the cat, but that wasn't enough to reverse the inflammation.

We started treating Helena with inhaled steroid (an anti-inflammatory agent) and asked her mother to monitor her progress with a peak flow meter. Initially, her morning readings were around 170 L/min, but gradually with treatment rose to 300 L/min. At that point we were able to cut the dose of inhaled steroid in half.

In Helena's case, because allergy to cat dander was such a prominent part of her asthma, by giving up the cat and treating the inflammation it was possible to reverse the course of her disease. In future, whenever she does develop an upper respiratory infection, she can use the bronchodilator for symptomatic relief and inhaled steroid to clear the inflammation.

Jonathan developed asthma as an infant. Each time he had a cold, he would experience a rapid onset of severe symptoms and end up in hospital. He also was a very allergic youngster, with allergies to egg and to peanut.

Jonathan constantly had symptoms of asthma, despite the use of an anti-inflammatory agent and at least two bronchodilators. Every time he got a cold, he would very quickly have an escalation of symptoms and develop a poor response to the inhaled bronchodilator.

We needed to use a stronger anti-inflammatory—a steroid—to treat Jonathan's severe asthma, but at the time it was not possible to administer inhaled steroid to a toddler. This meant that the only option was oral prednisone, but his parents worried about the side effects and did not want to use that option. Jonathan's asthma continued to be very severe. At age five, he had such a severe episode that he had to be admitted to an intensive care unit where he was on a respirator for a few days.

His parents then agreed to the prednisone and now give it to him as soon as he seems to be developing a cold. They monitor his lung capacity daily with a peak flow meter and keep close watch on his asthma, yet it is unstable despite the continuous use of high-dose inhaled steroid.

Sonny also developed asthma in infancy and was hospitalized several times. The anti-inflammatory Intal and several bronchodilators could not keep him out of trouble. His parents allowed the use of prednisone and would start it as soon as he showed signs of developing a cold. He was put on inhaled steroids as soon as the methods for administering them to young children became available. He is doing much better now. His asthma has become milder, although it is still at a level where he requires low-dose inhaled steroid daily to maintain a symptom-free state.

These last two patients are drawn from the severe end of the spectrum to illustrate the effectiveness of early, aggressive treatment. Children with such severe asthma represent less than 5 per cent of our patients. Fortunately, most children have milder asthma that can respond well to the mild, anti-inflammatory properties of sodium cromoglycate (see page 56).

Martin, the little boy we told you about at the beginning of this chapter, was treated more recently than Jonathan and Sonny. With him we were able to use the newer device, the pediatric mask aerochamber, which allows us to give inhaled medication by puffer to young children.

Our final case illustrates how treacherous asthma can become when it is not properly managed.

Peter was a thirty-four-year-old man who had had asthma since he was eighteen months of age. Throughout his childhood, symptoms had been fairly mild and he had obtained relief as needed from a bronchodilator. But when he reached his twenties, he had a few severe episodes requiring hospitalization. His doctor recommended he now start inhaled steroids, but Peter was hesitant. Instead he chose to follow the advice of an alternative therapist who recommended "natural" treatments. Although Peter followed the therapist's advice, avoided many chemicals and foods and even took "neutralizing drops" under his tongue, his asthma worsened. He had to use the bronchodilator daily, and still he would awaken in the night with sudden episodes of tightness. These were interpreted as sudden allergic episodes and he was given adrenaline and oxygen.

As his disease progressed, he had to give up exercising

and avoid even minimal exertion, but still he didn't improve. One night, the bronchodilator wasn't enough to relieve the congestion. Peter became unconscious and could not be revived.

This case reminds us that asthma can kill. We didn't include it to frighten you, but to point out the seriousness of the disease and the need for adequate medical treatment. With such treatment, 80 to 90 per cent of asthmatics can achieve complete freedom from all symptoms, even the mildest, by using safe amounts of medication. With others, like Jonathan, we aim for optimal control with minimum side effects from the medication.

CHAPTER FOUR

Hay Fever

At the mention of allergies, most people think of hay fever and immediately visualize an itchy runny nose, sneezing and red watery eyes. It is a common problem affecting 20 to 30 per cent of the population to some degree. Canadians spend an estimated $50 million annually on medications to clear their noses and relieve their symptoms.

WHAT IS HAY FEVER (RHINITIS)?

Actually, the term hay fever is a misnomer. Hay doesn't cause these symptoms, but during the hay-gathering season—mid-August to mid-September—pollen from ragweed is abundant in the air. For many people, this pollen starts the sequence of events that results in the nasal symptoms. Goldenrod, which many people associate with hay fever, is not as much of a problem as ragweed, since the pollen from goldenrod isn't carried as easily by the wind. We prefer the term **rhinitis** to describe the inflammation in the nose and the associated symptoms of itching and discharge.

The nose, sinuses and eyes

Although generally taken for granted, the nose is actually a delicate organ with important functions—filtering dirt particles from the air you breathe and warming and humidifying the air before it reaches your lungs. In your nose are sensory cells that give a sense of smell, and smell is an integral part of taste.

Linked to the nose by narrow channels are air-filled cavities, called sinus cavities. These lighten the skull and add resonance to your voice. Mucosal tissue, containing mast cells, lines both the nose and the sinus cavities.

The conjunctiva, a membrane that covers the white part of the eye and lines the inside of the eyelids, is also mucosal tissue. Thus swelling, itching, redness and tearing can occur in the eyes as well, with or without the nasal symptoms.

As we discussed in Chapter 1, for certain people, pollens can be the antigens that trigger an IgE-mediated immune response. The resulting inflammation in the mucosal tissues that line your nose and nasal passages causes the hallmarks of the disease—intense itching, swelling and leaking of copious amounts of clear, watery discharge.

This inflammation can also have non-allergic causes, but once it's present, the nasal passages become particularly sensitive to all sorts of other stimuli or irritants, such as sudden changes in the weather, strong smells and air pollution.

Allergic rhinitis

When diagnosing allergic rhinitis, we usually differentiate between the seasonal variety, which occurs during the spring, summer or fall, and perennial rhinitis, which occurs year-round. Although the symptoms are the same, the allergens that stimulate an IgE response are different. The inciting agents for seasonal rhinitis are tree, grass and weed pollens and outdoor mould spores. Perennial rhinitis is a response to house dust, animal dander and indoor moulds. Adult sufferers are more likely to have the perennial form, while children and teenagers usually have the seasonal problem. However, there can be considerable overlap.

The hallmarks of allergic rhinitis are:

- **An itchy nose.** If intense itching isn't present, we would wonder if the person really does have an allergy problem. To relieve the itching, a young child may rub against the bed sheets or develop rabbit-like movements of the nose. The "allergic salute" is another common habit—the child rubs a palm upward against the tip of the nose to relieve some itching and at the same time to elevate the nose slightly to allow for better passage of air through the nasal passages. An "allergic crease" may develop across the bridge of the nose where it is constantly wrinkled by rubbing.
- **Sneezing.** The congestion triggers bouts of vigorous sneezing, which can be very exhausting.
- **Nasal discharge.** The nose runs frequently with a clear, watery discharge. This distinguishes rhinitis from an infection, as then the discharge becomes thick and discoloured.

  During the night, the nasal discharge tends to drip into the back of the throat, causing irritation and dryness. The person may awaken with a hoarse voice and dry cough. (Note: A constant cough during the allergy season may also be a sign of asthma.)

- **Nasal congestion.** With the lining of the nose swollen, normal breathing becomes difficult. Because of this, mouth breathing is common, leading to a scratchy throat and dry lips, as the inhaled air isn't humidified.

  Snoring, a common habit in mouth breathers, may disturb sleep. In fact, many people find rhinitis leaves them constantly tired.

  Nasal congestion also interferes with the senses of smell and taste, and constant irritation and rubbing can cause frequent nose bleeds. In children, the prolonged obstruction and mouth breathing can stimulate an overgrowth of the upper jaw (overbite) and elongation of the face.

  The sinus cavities are also swollen, and the pressure in the sinuses causes headaches. "Allergic shiners," or dark circles under the eyes, develop because the blood flow in this area is slower.

  As people with rhinitis know only too well, the disease doesn't stay localized in the nose. Itchy, red, weepy eyes are very common as the allergen sets off an immune response in the conjunctiva. Some people also complain of buzzing or fullness in their ears, or occasional hearing problems. This is likely because the Eustachian tubes, which link the nose and ears, become blocked and cause pressure on the ears.

  As a consequence of the continued congestion, the nose, sinuses and ears may be more susceptible to infection; bacteria that become trapped in the sinus cavity can multiply and cause an infection.

Non-allergic rhinitis

Rhinitis can also occur when there is no evidence of an allergic cause; patients have negative skin tests.

In one kind of non-allergic rhinitis, eosinophils, a type of white blood cells, are recruited into the nasal area during the onset of inflammation. It is thought that these cells are important in maintaining the inflammation. People who have these eosinophils in their nasal discharge have a tendency to develop sinus disease and nasal polyps (growths in the nose) and are also more likely to be asthmatic. For these people, environmental factors such as humidity and temperature changes, pollution, smoke, chemical odours and pungent food smells, especially from spices, can worsen their problems. These people respond well to some of the medications we use in the treatment of allergic rhinitis.

Infectious rhinitis, caused by a virus or bacterial infection, is characterized by nasal congestion and a thick, cloudy, greenish nasal discharge. Sinusitis, which is an infection of the sinuses, may accompany such rhinitis. If any of these infectious diseases occurs repeatedly, your doctor may look for other causes, such as enlarged adenoids, structural birth defects or antibody-deficiency diseases.

There is a rare condition in which the cilia, the hairs in the nose, do not function properly so the person has difficulty fighting off infections.

Structural defects in the nose, such as nasal septal deviation, polyps, tumors and swollen adenoids, can also cause rhinitis. In children, polyps are more likely a sign of cystic fibrosis, and this needs to be ruled out.

Rhinitis may also be the result of a child lodging some

object, such as a crayon, in his nose. In this situation the discharge may become foul smelling and bloody.

Overuse of decongestant nose drops, ASA-containing medications (such as Aspirin), certain blood-pressure lowering drugs and cocaine can also cause nasal inflammation. In some adults, ASA sensitivity and nasal polyps may combine with perennial rhinitis to cause significant nasal congestion.

Nasal congestion is more common during pregnancy, but tends to clear after delivery.

Investigation of rhinitis

After asking about your symptoms and medical history, and examining your nose, your doctor will have a good idea whether to suspect allergies or other problems. Sinus and adenoid x-rays, as well as certain blood tests, can help rule out some of the non-allergic problems we've discussed. If allergy is the likely cause, skin testing or RAST measurement will help determine possible allergens.

MANAGEMENT OF RHINITIS

Whenever sensitivity to certain allergens is discovered, avoidance should be part of the management strategy. As with asthma, once the tissues are inflamed, regardless of whether the initial cause is allergy or not, many things in your environment can worsen the problem. You should use many of the strategies described in the next chapter to avoid pollens and tobacco smoke, regulate the humidity and temperature in your home, and reduce dust and animal dander.

Allergy shots

Allergy shots, or immunotherapy, commonly used in the past, are no longer necessary for most patients, now that we understand more about rhinitis and have safe, effective medications.

Immunotherapy consists of a series of injections of specific allergens. Small doses are given at first, and, if they are tolerated, successive larger doses are given to stimulate the production of protective antibodies by the body. This is done a short time before the individual's "allergy season." It would work if you were allergic to only one or two pollens and effective extracts were available for those pollens. Most extracts used in the past were very crude, however, and doctors had to resort to a "shotgun approach," with a mixture of many allergens in low doses given for many years. In many cases, when it did seem to work, it was probably because the child outgrew the allergies.

If tests have proven you're allergic to only one or two things, immunotherapy might be worth a one- or two-year trial. But if it isn't successful by then, give it up. (In Chapter 9, we will be discussing an appropriate use for immunotherapy with allergies to stinging insects.)

Allergy shots for hay fever are inconvenient for the patient, expensive and can be traumatic for children.

Since allergy shots for rhinitis are cumbersome and slow to be effective, and complete avoidance often isn't possible, if you want to lead a normal life, your management strategy should include medication that can reverse the inflammation that is already there.

Rhinitis medications

Over the last decade, there have been major advances in our understanding of allergies and improvements in the safety of the medications available. We now have a wider choice of rhinitis medications to choose from, so we can now tailor our treatment recommendations to the individual case. But no matter which medications we use, there is one overriding principle—the sooner the medications are used to begin controlling the inflammation, the better will be your results. In other words, as with asthma, let's put out the fire at the first sign of sparks.

Antihistamines. Antihistamines block the action of histamine, one of the major mediators released during an allergic response. Therefore, to be most effective, they should be taken just before exposure to an allergen or at the start of the allergy season, although they are still somewhat beneficial after the symptoms have already started.

Until a few years ago, most of the available antihistamines tended to cause drowsiness, confusion and dizziness as a side effect, and thus were not safe to use if you intended to drive a car or operate machinery. They also could cause ringing in the ears, dry mouth, blurred vision and urinary retention. But there are some newer antihistamines that do not cause drowsiness (Seldane, Reactine, Claritin and Hismanal).

Antihistamines are relatively safe medications, so they are sold without prescription. Some people with very mild rhinitis find that occasional use of these medications is all they need, but with so many brands to choose from, it may take some time for your doctor to find the best one for you.

Decongestants. Local application of over-the-counter nose drops and sprays (Otrivin and Neo-Synephrine) may help to decrease severe swelling. But these products should be used for only a few days at a time. If used too often or too long, they eventually cause swelling of the nasal membranes and worsen your symptoms. Oral decongestants (Sudafed) can also help occasionally, but are not appropriate for prolonged use either.

Other nasal sprays. If those listed above don't work, your doctor can prescribe more effective medications to meet your particular needs.

Medication, such as **Atrovent**, effectively controls the discharge brought on by inhaling irritants such as hot foods, various spices and cold air.

Rynacrom, an anti-inflammatory spray similar in action to Intal (used for asthma), prevents the release of mediators. Therefore, it is best used just before the pollen season, although it would still be beneficial when used at other times as well.

Nasal steroids (Beconase, Vancenase, Rhinalar, Nasocort, Rhinocort and Flonase) are the most effective medications for reducing inflammation in both allergic and non-allergic rhinitis. You may not notice improvement for a few days, so for patients with seasonal symptoms, we like to start the medication a week before the expected pollen release. Side effects include some local irritation and nose bleeds. If this happens, your doctor may adjust the dosage or recommend that you rub petroleum jelly into your nostrils before using the spray. There are fewer side effects with steroid sprays than with oral steroid medications.

Rhinitis is annoying, but it is not life-threatening. Many people think of it as just one of those things they must put up with during the late summer and fall months. People who have an occasional day of discomfort may achieve all the relief they need from non-prescription medications. But if you find you use such products daily for more than a couple of weeks, this is a sign you may need more help. Also, whenever rhinitis interferes with your ability to concentrate at work or at school, or when you must stay home for a day or two, or when you can't sleep at night because of the congestion, it's time to do something. See your doctor or allergist and ask for more help.

CHAPTER FIVE

Avoidance Strategies

After reading about the medical treatment of asthma and hay fever in the previous two chapters, you may be wondering if avoiding allergens and irritants is worth the bother. Even though complete avoidance is often impossible to achieve, improving your personal environment can help reduce the amount of medication you need. Most patients are able to achieve some reasonable balance between avoidance and a normal lifestyle.

This chapter is divided into three sections—home, work and school. But you'll want to read all three, as many strategies apply in all situations.

IMPROVING YOUR HOME ENVIRONMENT

Since you likely spend more than half of your time indoors, reducing the number of irritants in your home is a good place to start. You or your child may have lived in this environment for several years without problems, but, as we described in Chapter 1, you must first become sensitized to an allergen before you will notice any symptoms. Once sensitized, repeated exposures to the allergen cause the lining of nose or lungs to stay constantly inflamed.

In addition, once you have a twitchy nose or airways as a result of the inflammation, you are supersensitive to other airborne allergens, as well as many common environmental irritants, such as smoke or chemical smells. Any of these may escalate your problems, causing excess mucus, stuffiness, sneezing, coughing or difficult breathing. Even abrupt changes in temperature or weather can bring on an attack of asthma.

It is difficult to predict what will cause problems for a particular person. We can test for the usual allergens— pollens, dust mites or animal dander, but we can't tell you what combination of other things in your environment will create problems. Reactions are often a result of a combination of irritants acting in a snowball fashion. A child who has developed an allergy to ragweed pollen, for instance, is much more likely to react to the irritation from dust and smoke during that season. Even your current state of health is important. For example, smoke from the fireplace or cigarettes may bother you only when you have a viral cold.

Determining the cause of your problems is doubly difficult when your reactions are delayed. You might not notice the symptoms until an hour or two after exposure to smoke or a cat. But continued exposure can lead to chronic or worsening problems. This chapter suggests ways to reduce the level of all potential allergens and irritants in your home:

- house dust
- mould

- animals and birds
- pollens
- tobacco and fireplace smoke
- chemical irritants
- plant allergens

For children, the home environment is especially important. They spend more time there, particularly in their bedrooms, and their allergies tend to be more severe. Since the tendency to allergies is inherited, anything atopic parents can do to make their baby's or child's environment as allergen-free as possible can delay or perhaps decrease the severity of potential allergy problems.

> *Over the winter when Johnny was two, he was admitted to hospital several times because of acute bouts of asthma. During the last admission, he spent several days in the intensive care unit. That's when his father decided to make some changes at home. He gave away the cat, ripped out the wall-to-wall carpeting and improved the ventilation system. Since then, Johnny has been much healthier. His father has noticed a definite improvement, and although Johnny still has bouts of wheezing when he has a cold, he hasn't had to return to hospital since.*

Dr. Andrew Murray and his colleagues in British Columbia recently did a comparative study with twenty children known to be allergic to dust mites. Half the families were taught how to modify the children's bedrooms to make them as easy to clean as a hospital room. In one month, wheezing in the children with the easy-to-clean bedrooms dropped from 27 per cent to 2 per cent of the time. The need for medication also fell, from 30 per cent to 2 per cent. Other families who didn't make any changes in their homes did not see an improvement in their children.

Other studies have shown that dust mites in the home can increase the chance of asthma attacks sevenfold. Asthmatics living in the New Guinea Highlands, well away from industrial pollution, have a very high incidence of asthma. This is felt to be because their homes and climate are perfect for breeding dust mites.

Studies on cat allergens show that dander can remain suspended in the air for long periods of time, especially in homes where air circulation is poor. Controlling the home environment is an essential component of allergy management.

Establishing the cause
You can suspect there are problems in your home if:

- Symptoms suggestive of allergies, such as nose, eye, chest or skin problems are increasing in severity or frequency.
- More than one family member is suffering. Remember, allergies tend to run in families.
- Symptoms improve when you're outside, on vacation, or away from home for several hours.
- Symptoms started shortly after changes in your home, such as painting, remodeling, insulating, purchasing new appliances or starting new hobbies, or after you moved to a new house.
- Problems seem to be worse in certain areas of the house, such as the bedroom, basement or kitchen, or in areas of the house where there are unusual smells, leaks or dampness.

- Symptoms worsen at certain times of the year, such as when the furnace is first turned on.

When trying to determine which things in your environment are causing your problems, it is helpful to keep a diary of all the times you had symptoms. Note where you were when the symptoms started, what you were doing, how you were feeling before and what the weather was. Remember, problems often occur as a result of a combination of irritants, such as having a cold and being exposed to smoke.

The number of changes you need to make in your home will depend upon the severity of symptoms in your family. We realize that many families don't want to give up a family pet. If the allergy is mild, it may be sufficient to just ensure that the allergic person doesn't go near the pet often or let it into the bedroom. Also the pet should be washed every couple of weeks.

We also believe there isn't any sense in undertaking major home renovations if there is a chance they won't help. Recently we had a patient whose family had spent $100,000 refurbishing their home—installing a new ventilation system, new insulation, new flooring, etc.—to make it as environmentally clean as possible. We believe that was overkill.

Usually it isn't necessary to strip your home completely. Meticulous cleaning may be all that's necessary. However, if your house has defects in the construction, heating, cooling or ventilation systems that allow high levels of irritants or chemicals to build up, then some changes may be necessary. Later in this chapter, we will suggest which mechanical devices may help and which are useless. Before incurring major expenses, be sure the changes will be beneficial.

Steps to improve your home environment

Smoke control. Let's start with the most obvious pollutant—cigarette smoke. We're always amazed at families who worry about urea formaldehyde insulation but are unaware that their own smoking habits are filling the air with formaldehyde, nitrogen oxides and carbon monoxide—three of the four most hazardous airborne gases. Repeated studies have shown that children exposed to second-hand tobacco smoke are more likely to develop throat and chest infections, whether allergic or not. In a recent study done in Hamilton, Ontario, researchers compared the asthma problems of children living close to the town steel mill with those of children living quite far away. The severity of asthma was the same in both groups and correlated more with smoking in the home, especially by the mother, than with the home location. In light of this, if someone in your family has allergies, smoking should be forbidden in the home and in the family car.

In addition, you carry tobacco-smoke irritants on your clothes and in your hair to such a degree that limiting smoking to outside won't entirely solve the problem. Having an allergic child is good motivation to give up smoking entirely.

Fireplaces and wood stoves are another source of smoke irritants. For the sake of the comfort of the allergic member of your family, you may have to forgo romantic fireside evenings.

Dust control.   House dust harbours a complex mixture of many common allergens—dust mites, mould spores, animal dander, debris from furniture, food remnants, insect particles and pollen—but it is the dust mite that is the major allergy-causing component. Since these microscopic creatures feed on dead skin cells from humans and animals, they tend to collect in mattresses, chairs and couches, and carpets. They multiply most quickly when the temperature is about 25°C and the humidity is more than 50 per cent. Mites die when the temperature drops below 10°C, but a dead mite is still a problem since the mite feces and body parts are the main culprits.

It's hard to predict how much house dust you can tolerate. We recommend you start by removing all dust collectors from the bedroom, where you spend at least a third of your day. From there, you can decide if major changes in the rest of the house will help.

> **Dust mite particles fall quickly, so air filters won't help in removing them, but cleaning will.**

- **Keep humidity down**. Don't locate bedrooms in the basement where humidity tends to be higher. Buy a hygrometer (available in hardware stores), so that you can monitor the humidity level in bedrooms. Then, if necessary, you can use a portable dehumidifier in the bedroom or in rooms that tend to be damp. If you're buying such a unit, choose one with a capacity greater than 14 L, and empty it daily. Air conditioners help reduce humidity and house temperature in the summer. (For more on mechanical equipment, see page 96.)

- **Remove carpets**. Even daily vacuuming fails to remove all the dust mite particles from carpets, especially shag or wool ones. The mites have sucking pads on their legs, which help them to cling to carpet pile. Bare wood or linoleum floors are easier to clean effectively by washing, so pull out the wall-to-wall carpets, particularly in the bedroom. If you'd like a rug near the bed, choose a small, easily washed synthetic throw rug.

  If you want some carpeting in other parts of the house, choose short-pile carpets made of synthetic materials, and be sure the underpad is made of synthetic material. Vacuum the carpet often.

  Once or twice a year have your carpets professionally steam cleaned. Home rug-shampoo treatments tend to leave a chemical residue.

- **Vacuum thoroughly**. Dust easily escapes from some vacuum cleaners, especially the upright ones. A canister vacuum with a fresh disposable bag and a clean filter over the air vent is better. Take the vacuum cleaner outside to change the bag. If you have the choice, a central vacuum system with an outdoor exhaust is the best way to clean carpets.

- **Remove dust collectors**. Reduce the clutter typical of a child's room by removing chalk boards, cork boards, pennants, mobiles, hanging plants and open shelves. Keep toys and books in a closed box, drawer or cabinet—or, better yet, out of the bedroom completely. Beware of fuzzy, stuffed animals that can't be machine washed. If your child has a favourite stuffed animal, remove the stuffing and replace it with nylon stockings.

- **Put clothes away**. Put clothes away in a closet or drawers. If possible, store rarely used and out-of-season clothes away from the bedroom.
- **Choose appropriate bedding**. All bedding must be washable. Use synthetic or cotton blankets and bedspreads. Don't use quilts, comforters or eiderdowns, as they are harder to launder effectively. Recent studies suggest electric blankets, although more difficult to clean, reduce dust mites by lowering the humidity.

  Wash the sheets weekly, and all the bedding, including mattress covers and blankets, at least once a month in very hot water. Dry them in an automatic dryer, because if you hang them outside they could collect pollen.

  Use synthetic pillows, not ones stuffed with kapok, feathers or down. Foam pillows should be cleaned monthly as they tend to collect moulds.

  Since mattresses harbour many dust mites, encase both the mattress and box spring completely in plastic and seal with tape. Vacuum this cover when you change the sheets. Check for and seal any tears in the plastic. To prevent skin irritation when sleeping, use a polyester mattress pad or several sheets doubled over. Wash these often. A water bed is a good alternative to a conventional mattress, as it is easy to clean.

  Don't put canopies over beds. If you have bunk beds, give the upper bunk to the allergic child, and locate it away from any air vents, which tend to circulate dust.
- **Decorate simply**. Walls and ceilings are best painted or covered with a washable, flat-surface wallpaper. Avoid dust-collecting venetian blinds or shutters on

the windows. Instead, use short, light, untextured, easily washable curtains of Dacron or Terylene. If necessary, use roll-up window blinds for room darkening.

Keep just a minimum amount of wood, metal, vinyl or plastic furniture in the bedroom—none of it stuffed or upholstered. All fabrics, rugs, bedding and furniture become a problem after prolonged use and should eventually be discarded. If you have a mattress or box spring that is more than ten years old, throw it out.

- **Clean effectively**. Although the allergic member of the family should help in putting away toys, books and clothes, that person has a good excuse not to participate in regular cleaning. In fact, it's best if the person with allergies stays out of the room for several hours after cleaning as the level of airborne dust will be higher then.

  Damp mop or vacuum bedroom floors and furniture at least twice a week and, if possible, every day during the allergy season. Don't use dry cloths, mops or brooms as they just tend to spread the dust rather than remove it. Be sure you clean under and behind the mattress, box spring and all furniture at least once a month. Wash ceilings, windows, walls and baseboards at least three or four times a year. For routine cleaning avoid using strong solutions, such as Lysol or some of the lemon-scented cleaners, which can leave irritating chemical odours. Good substitutes are vinegar and water or baking soda and water.

  After cleaning, if you want to air the room, do it in the middle of the day, when the pollen count is lowest and when the person with allergies is out of the room.

Then close the windows and doors for an hour or so before the allergic person returns to the room.

Some mite-killing chemicals are now being developed and may soon be available for reducing dust mite levels.

Mould control. Moulds or mildew are types of fungus that live off decaying plant life. They give off spores, which can become airborne, and thus inhaled by a sensitive person.

Moulds can live year-round in your home. They flourish in dark, damp places, or wherever the humidity is above 50 per cent. Outside, they're a problem from spring to fall in any place that is damp, such as rotting vegetation and leaves. On hot, dry, windy days or after a rainfall, the spores are readily

> To keep the dust mites and moulds from multiplying, keep your house temperature between 20 and 21°C, and the humidity between 25 and 40 per cent.

dispersed through the air. Although it's impossible to avoid exposure to moulds completely, check the places listed in the table on pages 90–91 for places that attract moulds.

Anything you can do to reduce humidity both throughout the house and in the pockets of moisture in certain areas will help in reducing mould growth in your home. Many of the measures suggested previously for dust mite control will help to reduce moulds, but in addition:

- Wash surfaces such as window ledges and shower stalls with Lysol or chlorine bleach at least once every

---

Places moulds will accumulate

Outdoors:
- freshly mown grass
- piles of leaves
- composters and compost heaps
- areas of poor drainage
- wood piles
- hay stacks, grain bins
- garbage cans
- camping equipment—sleeping bags, tents, boat cushions
- lawn mowers
- golf bags
- cars—under the floor mats or in the air-conditioning system

Indoors:
- recently opened cottages, hotels and motels
- unfinished basements

---

three months. These cleaners are very effective at killing moulds, but they do release irritating fumes. Therefore, use them only for special cleaning, rinse well and air the chemical fumes from the room before the allergic person returns.
- Use mould-resistant paint on walls in unfinished basements.
- Use dehumidifiers, but be sure to clean them weekly.
- Clean other ventilation equipment and replace filters often in furnaces, air conditioners and dehumidifiers. Disinfect vaporizers before using.

- crawl spaces and attics
- utility rooms
- shower stalls and soap dishes
- cracks between bathroom tiles
- shower curtains
- magazines left in the bathroom
- refrigerator coils or drip trays
- window mouldings
- aquariums
- soil around potted plants
- air conditioners, dehumidifiers, humidifiers and vaporizers
- furnace filters
- damp closets
- damp shoes and boots
- surfaces soiled by children or pets
- foods and food cupboards—especially dried fruit, vegetables, old bread, aged cheese, pickled foods, beer, wine, vinegar and soy sauce

- Minimize house plants or cover the soil with plastic wrap. Nurseries also sell mould-inhibiting solutions you can add to the soil.
- Keep aquariums out of the bedrooms altogether. If you have one in another room, keep it small.
- Cover the ground in crawl spaces with black polyethylene sheets. Install drains that effectively remove standing water.
- Use exhaust fans, vented to the outside, after bathing or when cooking or laundering to remove water vapours.

- In damp closets, leave on a low-wattage light bulb as a heat source, or store some hygroscopic crystals on the top shelf, out of reach of children.
- Increase the sunlight in your yard by trimming or cutting down trees and shrubs.

Animal control. The animals that affect allergic people include house pets—cats, dogs, birds, gerbils, guinea pigs, hamsters, rabbits—as well as farm animals such as horses and sheep. Animals have dander (skin scales) and birds have both dander and feathers, which can cause allergic reactions. Small, non-shedding animals can cause as many allergy problems as larger, long-haired animals, as it is the dander, not the hair, that is the problem. A person may also be sensitive to urine from guinea pigs and a component in the saliva of dogs and cats. When an animal grooms, it deposits this saliva on its hair.

> **There are no "non-allergenic" cats and dogs. All have dander, as do rabbits, guinea pigs and even birds.**

Removing the animal from your home is the best course of action. Even then, it will take from three to six months before all the dander disappears. Professional cleaning of the carpets and air ducts will help speed up the process.

If you cannot part with the family pet, establish the following house rules:

- The animal stays out of the bedrooms.
- The allergic person doesn't wash the pet, although pets should be washed every week or two, as this helps remove some dander.
- The animal stays outside as much as possible.

- The pet doesn't enter tents or cabins where you may be sleeping.
- The pet doesn't go on car trips with the allergic person.
- When the pet dies, it will not be replaced.

Other ways to help the person with animal allergies:

- Encourage family members and visiting friends who have close contact with an animal to change their clothes before entering your house.

  We had a very young patient who, on testing, reacted to horse dander. She'd never been to a farm or near horses, but her father was a veterinarian.

- Take an antihistamine or asthma medication before visiting a home where there are animals. If you're going to be staying overnight, the pet should be kept out of the room, the bedding changed and the room thoroughly cleaned.
- Ask teachers not to keep any animals in the classroom (see alternative suggestions on pages 105 and 106).

Chemical control.   Many of the products we use around the home on a daily basis—paints, perfumes, insecticides, hairsprays, deodorants, cleaning agents, waxes and glues—contain chemicals that give off irritating or allergy-producing vapours. It may take some detective work to determine which of these bother the allergic member of your family. Thus, the more you can do without these products, the better.

   Often you can find a safer alternative:

- stick, non-perfumed deodorants

- baking soda, washing soda or vinegar solutions for cleaning walls, kitchens and bathrooms
- baking soda as an air freshener

Alternative Home Cleaners is a free pamphlet of tips and recipes for cleaners based on vinegar, pure soap, baking soda, borax and ammonia that is available from Pollution Probe, 12 Madison Ave., Toronto, Ontario, M5R 2S1. However, don't use the ammonia in the home of a person with allergies.

Whenever you use cleaning materials or paints, keep the windows open or use ventilation fans if you have them. When finished, seal the containers and store them well away from the bedrooms.

Many building materials contain chemicals that give off noxious gases. Urea formaldehyde is perhaps the best-known example, but caulking compounds, sealants, solvents, glass fibres and fire retardants in cellulose can cause problems for some people with allergies. It's best for the allergic person to stay away during any home renovations.

Pollutants in incoming air.   Even the most energy-efficient homes will have a complete change of air every five hours of so. Therefore, it's important to think about the quality of outside air that may be entering your home. Check for odours in rooms adjacent to or above an attached garage. There may be leaks through which car exhaust fumes or fumes from stored chemicals enter. Position any outside vents from kitchen, bathroom and dryers as high as possible so that exhaust fumes do not recirculate into the home. Reduce the amount of outdoor air pollution that enters your home by closing windows during peak exposure times, such as the morning and evening traffic rush.

Workplace irritants—such as wood dust, cotton dust and chemical fumes—can also enter the home on the clothes of family members. Anyone who works in an environment where there is frequent exposure to chemical irritants should wash and change clothes immediately after work.

Pollen control. Pollen from trees, grass and weeds is light enough to be carried by the wind, but also light enough to be inhaled. It can easily enter the home through open windows and on the clothes of family members. In Canada, trees pollinate in early spring, grasses in late spring and early summer and ragweed in late summer and early fall. The amount of pollen in the air depends on the weather and wind conditions and hence varies from year to year and place to place. Pollen counts reported on radio and in the newspaper tend to be general and for a wide area. They may not be accurate for around your home.

Although you can't control pollen outside, you can reduce the amount that comes into your home with the following measures:

- Keep windows closed as much as possible. (This helps in cars, as well.)
- Use an air conditioner or effective furnace filtering system. (See pages 98 and 99.)
- Avoid planting trees and shrubs close to the house, especially near the bedroom windows.
- Keep your garden as weed-free as possible.

- During the spring, summer and fall, remove and launder clothes after they've been worn outside for gardening or playing in the grass.

Unusual plant allergens.   Without realizing it, you may be bringing some products containing allergy-producing plant components into your home.

Pyrethrum, an extract from dried chrysanthemum-related plants, is often in insecticides and even flea-fighting pet shampoos and collars. A person who is sensitive to ragweed may react to pyrethrum.

Kapok, another plant allergen, comes from the seed pods of the kapok tree. Because it is water-resistant, it is often used in sleeping bags, boat cushions, life jackets, boots—and is even found in antique furniture.

Some mattresses and furniture upholstery contain **cottonseed** (unrefined cotton) and **cotton linters** (short fibres from cotton seeds), which are common allergens. The refined cotton used in sheets and clothes is not a problem. Cottonseed is also used in fertilizers, animal feeds and baked goods. Cottonseed flour can be highly allergenic when eaten or inhaled, although cottonseed oil is usually not a problem.

MECHANICAL DEVICES FOR ENVIRONMENTAL CONTROL

If any member of your family is hospitalized often or needs several kinds of medication to control the allergy, then it's time to consider a complete overhaul of your home. Some filtering devices are sold with promises that they will clean the air and provide welcome relief for allergy sufferers. Although some are worthwhile, many are a waste of money. Be very sure the device will be helpful before you open your pocketbook. The *Canadian Consumer* and *Consumer Reports* magazines have some of the best evaluations of these products. You can find the magazines in your local library.

Humidifiers. When your home is too dry (humidity that's below 25 per cent), tiny cracks may develop in your nose and respiratory tract, making it easier for allergens to irritate and for infections to start. Conversely, moulds, dust mites and fungi multiply rapidly when the humidity is high. The ideal humidity level is between 25 and 40 per cent.

Humidifiers can be helpful during Canadian winters when the inside air is too dry, but these units can also become an ideal harbour for moulds, bacteria and fungi. If you don't clean the unit before turning it on, you will be releasing the moulds into the air.

Central humidifiers attached to the furnace are helpful, but for best results at maintaining a constant level of humidity in the bedroom of the allergy sufferer, we recommend, in addition, a self-regulating portable unit. In general, a portable humidifier is easier to clean and you should do this every few weeks. Use chlorine bleach and a scrub brush, then rinse well to remove the chemical residue before turning it on again. Replace the filters more often than the manufacturer recommends. You'll find that if you use demineralized or distilled water, you have less accumulation of dust-collecting scale.

Vaporizers and so-called cold humidifiers do not turn off automatically when the humidity exceeds the ideal level. Therefore, we don't recommend them for regulating humidity on a daily basis. However, they may be useful for occasional relief of a congested nose. For that purpose, the cool-mist vaporizers are more comfortable than the hot-mist ones. Ultrasonic humidifiers tend to be quieter and more efficient than the older cool-mist ones. They also accumulate less moisture. Be sure you disinfect the humidifier tank after each use and store it dry.

During the summer months, the problem is often the reverse—too much humidity, especially in basements. If the hygrometer reading exceeds 50 per cent, we recommend you use a portable dehumidifier with a minimum capacity of 14 L per day.

Heating systems.   Since dust mites thrive best at temperatures above 25°C, keep your home temperature between 20 and 21°C. There is no one ideal heating system for the allergic person. Forced-air heating is probably your least expensive option, but you'll have to be sure to clean the furnace filters weekly and replace them monthly during the heating season. Baseboard electrical heaters and hot-water radiators are not as effective at maintaining a uniform temperature throughout the room, and, since these tend to be dust collectors, you'll have to clean them often. Heat pumps may be very energy efficient, but they are not the best choice for the allergic person, as they will be constantly bringing in outside air laden with pollens or other chemical irritants.

Annually, before the heating season, hire a professional furnace-cleaning firm to vacuum all the duct work. Otherwise, you'll be constantly recirculating dust and dust mites.

In the bedroom, cover any vents with a portion of a standard furnace filter to block out dust. Be sure beds are not directly in line with the ducts.

Avoid kerosene heaters and wood or coal stoves, as the smoke, carbon monoxide, sulphur dioxide and other gases produced can significantly irritate a person with allergies. Any energy cost savings you might realize will be offset by the expense of proper installation and regular cleaning.

For air cooling, both central and portable air conditioners help, as they allow you to remain more comfortable when staying inside with the doors and windows closed on hot, humid days. They don't effectively clean the air, however, as they operate only intermittently, but they are helpful in reducing humidity.

Air cleaners. Despite advertising promises, portable air cleaners do not do an effective job at removing irritating particles from the air. Before you invest in one, try all the other dust-reducing procedures, because no filter can take the place of effective cleaning. Remember that, for the most part, mite antigens are heavy and fall quickly; therefore cleaning, rather than filters, is the most effective way to reduce them.

For other airborne antigens, the only worthwhile air cleaners are the High Efficiency Particulate Air (HEPA) filters; both central and portable units are available. To keep your HEPA air cleaner working effectively, you'll have to replace the filters once or twice a year. A major disadvantage with these units is that they are expensive.

There isn't any point in buying the small, desk-top air cleaners. They can do little but freshen the room. Larger units with mechanical filters remove only large particles that don't create allergy problems anyway. An electrostatic filter can remove smaller airborne particles, but in the process it releases ozone as a by-product. The ozone itself is an irritant for many people with allergies. Negative ion machines have no proven significant value for people with allergies.

IMPROVING YOUR WORK ENVIRONMENT

Buildings protect against the weather, but they don't necessarily protect against indoor air pollution. As Benjamin Franklin wrote, "No common air from without is so unwholesome as the air within a closed room that has been often breathed and not changed."

Allergic and asthmatic patients can experience a worsening of their symptoms as a result of constant exposure to irritants at work. Even people without allergies experience discomfort when spending long hours in polluted buildings.

In your home, you can exercise considerable control over your environment. But people with allergies also need to make employers aware of changes they can make to improve the quality of air for all workers. This shouldn't come as a surprise. After all, employers know that if the office temperature drops below 20°C or if it is too drafty, employees are less comfortable and less productive. Now they must also realize that if the office is stuffy or smoky, the workers will become sluggish. It is never easy to make changes, but everyone stands to benefit from reduced absenteeism and increased ability to work effectively.

With our current concern about energy costs, we are increasingly designing buildings to minimize air exchange. Windows are sealed so that air exchange can be mechanically regulated. Most modern office buildings recirculate 80 per cent of air, and some try to conserve energy, even more, by shutting down the heating, air conditioning and ventilation systems at night and over the weekend. Adding to indoor pollution is a host of synthetic building materials, furnishings and office equipment—such as asbestos ceiling tiles, urea formaldehyde insulation, carpet glue, paints and solvents, and window caulking—all of which can give off toxic fumes.

Current estimates suggest that 20 to 30 per cent of office employees regularly experience symptoms that probably reduce their working efficiency. The terms "tight building syndrome" and "sick building syndrome" have been coined to describe a variety of symptoms that include dry skin, headaches, fatigue and repeated patterns of nose, eye and throat irritation, which are believed to result from prolonged exposure to poor indoor air.

Common symptoms of building-related illnesses

- Itching or burning eyes
- Dry or irritated throat
- Rhinitis, sinus congestion, sneezing
- Cough, chest tightness
- Skin rashes
- Headaches
- Drowsiness, fatigue
- Confusion, irritability, difficulty concentrating
- Dizziness

Between 1971 and 1988, the National Institute of Occupational Safety and Health investigated approximately

450 complaints of building-related illnesses in the United States. They found the following problems:

- 52%   Inadequate ventilation. The building ventilation did not meet standards for minimum ventilation rates.
- 17%   Contamination from inside the building. Tobacco smoke, chemical odours from equipment solutions, and rug shampoos are common problems.
- 11%   Contamination from outside the building. Improperly located exhaust and intake vents, periodic changes in prevailing winds and exhaust fumes drawn in through the ventilation system from parking garages are common contributors.
- 5%   Microbial contamination. This included the rare and difficult-to-diagnose diseases of hypersensitivity pneumonitis and humidifier fever. (See page 103.)
- 3%   Contamination from building materials. Urea-formaldehyde foam and plywood can emit formaldehyde fumes. There can also be fibrous glass erosion from ventilation ducts, and chemical odours from glues, adhesives and silicon caulking.
- 12%   Unknown.

Steps to improve your work environment
Reduction of tobacco smoke.   In Canada, we are making some progress in reducing one of the worse indoor air pollutants—tobacco smoke. The concentration of irritating smoke in a room where someone is smoking far exceeds that caused by any emission from a polluting industry. Any person with airways already inflamed by allergies has good reason to want to avoid further irritation from second-hand smoke. Smoking should be banned, not only in areas where a person with allergies works, but also

throughout any sealed building, as energy-efficient heating and air-conditioning systems tend to recirculate warmed indoor air.

Effective heat and humidity control. Many people will remember the 1976 outbreak of Legionnaire's disease in Philadelphia, in which many members of the Legion of Veterans of the American Army developed a flu-like illness while attending a convention at a hotel. After much investigation, the cause of the illness was traced to bacteria in cooling towers located near the hotel's air-conditioning system.

All parts of a heating, ventilation and air-conditioning system—including ducts, fan coils, baffle plates, tanks and so on—can harbour microorganisms, such as fungi.

A syndrome called humidifier fever, or "Monday fever," is characterized by lethargy, headache, fever and sometimes coughing and breathlessness at the beginning of each week. Symptoms seem to improve during the week, but recur at the start of the next work week. Outbreaks such as these have occurred when humidifiers are contaminated by microorganisms. Remedies include:

- Locating air-cooling towers in places where their effluent is not sucked in again by the fans of the conditioning plant. In some buildings, the cause of illnesses has been traced to motor vehicle exhaust, diesel fumes and boiler gases trapped and recirculated indoors.
- Choosing a dry steam humidification system rather than cold-water spray humidifiers. The dry steam system is less likely to support bacterial contamination.

- Keeping humidity below 70 per cent to reduce rapid growth of microorganisms (ideal level is between 25 and 40 per cent).
- Ensuring that all duct work is regularly cleaned and filters replaced often.
- Mopping up liquid spills as quickly as possible.
- Ensuring that carpets are perfectly dry after they are shampooed.
- Covering the soil on office plants with plastic wrap to reduce fungus growth.
- Repairing or replacing mouldy window frames.

Effective ventilation.   In some offices, employees have experienced outbreaks of nonspecific rashes, intense itching over the uncovered parts of their body, as well as difficulty wearing contact lenses. In most instances, the cause was traced to ventilation ducts lined with glass fibre insulation that had been damaged during remodeling or by water leaks. The solution would be to repair the ducts to prevent glass fibres from becoming airborne.

Urea-formaldehyde insulation materials, melamine formaldehyde resins in drapes and carpets, solvents used for carpet adhesives, asbestos fireproofing in older buildings, detergent residues left in carpets after shampooing, developing solutions used in photocopying machines, even liquid ink erasing solutions can all contribute to toxic irritation in the office. This list doesn't even begin to deal with chemicals used in industrial processes. Since it is probably impossible to furnish a modern office without using at least some chemical materials, the solution must be adequate ventilation.

Unless the building is located in a heavily polluted

area, increasing the rate of air exchange will help dilute indoor-generated air pollutants. Even though heating or cooling this air is an added expense, increasing air exchange from 0.2 changes per hour to 0.8 changes per hour can improve air quality fourfold.

IMPROVING THE SCHOOL ENVIRONMENT

A significant proportion of the school population, 15 to 20 per cent, suffers from the diseases discussed in this book. Since these children attend school for significant lengths of time, anything that can be done to improve the environment at school will help the children feel better and therefore concentrate and learn more effectively.

All the strategies on dust, humidity and temperature control, adequate ventilation and choice of building materials and furnishings that we've outlined in the previous sections apply to schools as well. In addition, the classroom setting has some more items, such as animals and chalk dust, that aggravate the child's condition.

Children with allergies may not experience problems every day but if they have a cold or are otherwise stressed, then things like dust, air pollution, exercise and cold air may aggravate their condition. This is why we believe some of the following suggestions are important for teachers and school administrators.

- **Do not keep animals or pets in classrooms**. We recognize the teaching benefits of watching the daily activities of animals, but there are reasonable compromises. Keep the animals in a separate room where children can visit them regularly. The room chosen should have good ventilation, in order to remove as much of the odour as possible. Children with allergies might visit the animals for short periods, either daily or weekly. If necessary, they can don masks before entering the room. They may also need to take certain prescribed medications fifteen to twenty minutes before visiting the animal room.

- **Excuse allergic children from certain duties**, such as being chalk monitors or doing other chores that might generate dust. They can help in other ways.
- **Eliminate carpeting in classrooms.** Carpets can harbour dust mites and moulds, which are difficult to remove.
- **Keep plants in the classroom to a minimum.** The suggestions made for animals in the classroom can also apply to plants. If some plants must be kept in the room, cover the soil with plastic wrap so as to minimize exposure to the mould and dust found in soil.
- **Monitor the sharing of lunches and snacks.** This prevents a child with food allergies from eating the wrong food. If one child in the classroom has a severe peanut allergy that could result in death, advise all parents not to send sandwiches, cookies or cakes that contain peanut butter or peanuts. (See page 117.)
- **Ensure that the room is well ventilated.** This is particularly important when the class is painting or using other chemicals.
- **Monitor school construction and renovation.** Apply the points discussed earlier in this chapter on heating, ventilation and air conditioning and the wise choice of building materials.
- **Delay major renovations and painting until school holidays.**

Because teachers and school officials play such a key role in the child's development, there is much more that they can do to ease the life of a child with an allergic disease. Therefore, in Chapter 10 we will discuss some additional pointers for teachers. We hope all school personnel read these suggestions, because there is a good likelihood that at some time you will have an opportunity to help an allergic child.

CHAPTER SIX

Food Allergies

Foods are not as common allergens as you may think. Many people believe they are allergic to certain foods, when in fact other allergens may be the culprit—or the person may not even have an allergy problem. In a recent survey of twenty-three patients coming to an allergy clinic with suspected food allergies, tests proved that only four were actually allergic to certain foods.

When we hear of patients who avoid many foods and live on very limited diets, we suspect that their problems have not been properly diagnosed. People who focus on food as the cause of health problems sometimes miss noticing other possible causes such as weather changes, pollution or animal dander. In our practice, we see many infants with transient food allergies, some children with long-term food allergies, and many more whose parents think they have food allergies but who, when tested appropriately, don't have allergies at all.

> **People living on very restricted diets may be jeopardizing their nutritional status unnecessarily.**

UNDERSTANDING FOOD ALLERGIES

A common misconception is that atopic individuals tend to be allergic to many foods. A study at Johns Hopkins Medical School of people who had definite food allergies revealed that 70 per cent had a problem with just one or two foods, 19 per cent reacted to three foods and only 3 per cent reacted to four or more different foods. This research provided two additional important facts: the foods that were the real culprits were not necessarily the ones the patients were avoiding. Most food allergies are to just eight food categories—milk, wheat, soy, egg, peanut, nuts, fish and shellfish.

Food intolerances versus food allergies

There's a difference between a food allergy and a food intolerance. If a person is allergic to a food, he will react to even small amounts of the food, sometimes even the crumbs left on a knife. A person may be so sensitive to a food such as fish that he will feel mildly ill from simply smelling the food. Such severe allergies are rare. Many infants with food allergies do outgrow them, especially if the allergy is to milk or egg. Allergies to peanut, nuts and shellfish are more likely to persist.

Food intolerances, unlike allergies, are dose-specific. That is, a person may be able to tolerate small servings of a specific food, but experience symptoms, such as stomach cramps or diarrhea, with larger servings. There are several important food intolerances.

Lactose intolerance is a disease in which the person lacks a particular enzyme, lactase, which is needed for the digestion of the sugar in milk and certain milk products. This enzyme deficiency is common in certain races, particularly Asians. These people may experience vomiting, diarrhea and bloating after drinking a full glass of milk, but may be able to tolerate a little milk in coffee. A person with lactose intolerance can drink special milk in which the sugar has been predigested, that is, the lactose has already been broken down, whereas a person with a milk allergy must avoid all milk, even foods that contain milk protein, such as bread.

A person with **celiac disease**, another food intolerance, has a problem with the protein (gluten) in wheat and some other grains. This disease is probably due to an immune response to gluten, but not an allergic immune response.

Chemicals in certain foods can cause **drug-like intolerances**—caffeine found in coffee, tea and cola beverages is one example; phenylethylamine, a stimulant in chocolate, is another.

Some people experience **gustatory rhinitis**, which is a very runny nose when eating certain foods, particularly spicy foods such as chili peppers, horseradish, red cayenne pepper, hot sauce, onion, vinegar and mustard. This is a temporary condition that lasts only as long as the food is being eaten. Certain chemicals in the foods (such as capsaicin) are stimulating sensory nerves in the mouth and throat. The nerve response can also cause eye tearing, forehead perspiration and facial flushing. Unlike the usual allergic rhinitis, gustatory rhinitis is rarely accompanied by sneezing, congestion or intense itching; skin tests with extracts of the implicated foods are consistently negative.

None of these examples involves IgE antibodies, so none is a true allergic reaction.

Symptoms of food allergies

Food allergies can appear in different ways—hives; swelling in the eyes, face, lips, hands, feet and genitals; red, watery eyes; laboured breathing; coughing, wheezing, nasal itching and discharge; stomach cramps, nausea, vomiting and diarrhea. Occasionally, a person has a life-threatening reaction that we call **anaphylaxis**. This is a reaction in which the blood vessels expand rapidly in response to the mediators (see page 15). When this happens, the blood pressure may drop suddenly, causing the patient to collapse. Immediate medical help is needed or the person could die.

> **A true IgE-mediated food allergy has to be consistently associated with the ingestion of a particular food. It will occur soon after eating the food.**

Most true food allergies—that is, IgE-mediated reactions, occur immediately—within seconds, minutes or a few hours of eating the foods. Reactions that occur many hours or days after eating a particular food are not IgE-mediated and are likely due to other non-food related causes. Therefore it is unlikely that a food eaten the night before is responsible for symptoms the following morning.

A mother who thought that regular cow's milk might be causing her son's wheezing and stuffy nose switched to goat's milk. She thought he had improved and thus, in her mind, her suspicions were confirmed. Skin testing, however, did not indicate a cow's milk allergy. We pointed out to the mother that the improvement in the asthma symptoms occurred coincidentally with the start of summer. It could be that the improvement was due to the boy no longer having the frequent colds that were aggravating his asthma. We advised her to keep a careful diary of other environmental factors—not just foods—that could be related to asthma.

Diagnosis of food allergies
Sometimes it's easy to identify a food allergy. If a child's lips and face swell within minutes of eating peanuts, it is obvious that peanuts are the cause of an allergy. But other cases are more difficult, especially if the food is used as an ingredient in many other foods.

A common problem in diagnosing food allergies is that people tend to discount foods that have been eaten without incident in the past. But remember that a person must become sensitized through previous exposure before there will be an allergic reaction.

If the patient has been ill, especially with an infection in the bowel area, foods are more likely to cause problems, although some of these reactions are non-allergic in nature. It's not surprising, therefore, that some food allergies have been wrongly diagnosed, especially if the proper tests were not done.

After studying the patient's diet history, the doctor generally confirms his or her suspicions with a prick test, as described in Chapter 2. These skin tests are not as precise as we'd like them to be. They will not always match the patient's ability to tolerate or not tolerate a particular food. Foods that cause positive skin tests may actually be well tolerated by one patient, while another

> **Skin testing for food allergies is a guide, but it is not always 100 per cent predictable. The doctor must also consider the patient's symptoms along with the results of the skin test.**

patient will experience a clinical reaction to the given food. If the skin test is negative, most patients will usually be able to tolerate the particular food without a reaction. Only a small number of patients with negative skin tests have reactions to a food.

The following case illustrates the appropriate use and interpretation of skin testing.

> *Rajunan was first brought to our offices when he was seventeen months old. His parents said he'd been wheezing an average of twenty days a month ever since he was four months of age, yet there had never been an indication that he was allergic to any foods. His parents didn't think his symptoms were related to exposure to animals, although there was a cat at his day-care center.*
>
> *We tested him, using the prick method, and he developed a large positive reaction to both egg and cat dander. Since he tolerated egg well, it was not necessary to eliminate it from his diet. Rajunan's asthma was being aggravated by the cat dander.*

When skin testing is not appropriate, perhaps because the patient has eczema, or when the results are questionable, we can use the blood RAST measurement. If both the skin and blood tests prove inconclusive, the doctor might ask you to keep a food diary—a record of all foods eaten, how the foods were prepared and the nature and times of the onset of symptoms. A pattern will likely emerge.

When the answer is still not obvious, we may eliminate one or two foods from the diet to see if the patient improves. We then watch for the symptoms to return the next time the suspect food is eaten. It is not necessary to eliminate many foods at one time. We think that type of testing is overused, and we are concerned that too many children become malnourished as a result of staying on a very restricted diet for an unnecessarily long period of time.

To confirm a food allergy, the most reliable procedure is to use challenge testing as described on page 30. This must be done in the doctor's office or, in certain cases, in the hospital, where treatment can be given immediately, if necessary. If there has been a recent history of a life-threatening reaction, challenge testing should not be done. It may be considered, however, for the evaluation of past life-threatening reactions that the patient might have outgrown.

MANAGEMENT OF FOOD ALLERGIES

The only safe way to prevent a food allergy reaction is strict avoidance. Drugs such as sodium cromoglycate (Intal) and ketotifen (Zaditen) have been tried, but the results to date have been disappointing. Research to determine if patients can be desensitized to peanut allergy by injections of small doses of peanut is being tested, but whether this will be successful or not remains to be determined.

In the meantime, allergic individuals must avoid the foods that cause problems. That is relatively easy to do if you are allergic to a food like strawberries or chocolate. But if you are allergic to a basic food, such as milk or egg, which is commonly used as an ingredient in recipes or other food products, you may need help in planning a nutritionally balanced diet and finding alternatives. Ask for counselling from a qualified dietitian.

With food allergies, constant vigilance is necessary because food manufacturers may change the contents of their products. Ingredient labels can give clues, but people with allergies must know all the variations of an ingredient. For example, albumin, egg (white, yolk, dried, powdered, solids), egg substitutes, egg nog, mayonnaise and meringue all indicate the presence of egg protein. Mandalona can be ground peanut that has been moulded and flavoured to resemble an almond. More information on sources of common food allergens is available from the allergy associations listed on pages 205 and 206.

When you're eating out you must ask food handlers about the ingredients in a dish and even check the recipes of foods served at parties.

> *A young woman attending her friend's wedding joined in the celebration by eating a piece of wedding cake. She had inquired about the foods being served, but had not suspected that the marzipan icing contained peanut paste. Within minutes of eating the cake, she had a major anaphylactic reaction. Even though a doctor at the wedding tried to resuscitate her, it was too late.*

Peanut allergies

Peanut allergies are now the leading cause of food-induced, life-threatening (anaphylactic) responses. It has been estimated that peanut is 1,000 times stronger than milk in causing allergic reactions. In fact, an allergic child can react if he licks the residual peanut butter left after a table top is wiped clean. Even the vapours released when a sealed jar of peanut butter is first opened can cause breathing difficulties in severely allergic individuals.

The reason why peanut causes such severe reactions is a mystery. Peanuts are capable of inducing a major reaction on the first known exposure. It is thought that babies may become sensitized to peanut through breast milk.

The number of peanut-sensitive Canadians seems to be on the rise, possibly because peanut butter is such a popular food. In Japan, where more people eat rice, and in Sweden, where fish is a dietary staple, those foods are more common allergens.

> **Anaphylaxis is a life-threatening allergic reaction. The muscles around the airways may go into spasm, making it difficult to breathe; blood vessels expand rapidly causing a sudden drop in blood pressure, which may lead to unconsciousness and death.**

Pure peanut oil does not generally pose a threat to peanut-sensitive people because the protein has been destroyed. However, cold pressed peanut oil and peanut oil manufactured outside of North America may contain some peanut protein. Therefore, unless you can be sure of the purity of the oil, avoidance is the safest option.

People who are peanut sensitive should be very cautious about cross-contamination. If you buy nuts from open bins, be aware that they could become contaminated with peanut by someone who inadvertently used the scoop in the peanut bin. Similarly, ice cream or yogurt dispensed from a machine could contain bits of peanut from a previous customer's order.

Lunchroom Safety

Because of the possible seriousness of a peanut reaction, Canadian allergists stress the need for allergy-safe environments in schools. Their recommendations include:

- no sharing of food, utensils or containers
- handwashing before and after eating
- washing (not just wiping) table tops, toys, etc. that have been exposed to food
- not using food for play or crafts
- strict supervision of younger children during meals and snacktime to prevent swapping
- a complete ban on peanuts in nursery schools, and allergy-free classrooms in primary schools where there is an allergic child
- special training for school food handlers on what to look for on labels and how to avoid cross-contamination of foods. (Allowing only home-prepared food is safer, where possible.)

A complete ban on several foods in addition to peanut could be very difficult to implement. Thus, while it may be difficult to create an allergy-free environment, the cooperation of teachers, students and parents can go a long way towards creating an allergy-safe environment. Information on students' allergies should be readily accessible to all caregivers. Special care should be taken to ensure substitute teachers, volunteers and occasional caregivers have this information.

Despite precautions, accidental ingestions may still occur. Safety procedures need to be in place anywhere children gather for school or recreational activities. Adults who have life-threatening allergies should alert their friends, co-workers and relatives. Anyone with such an allergy should wear appropriate identification. (See page 159.)

In an emergency, immediate administration of epinephrine (adrenaline) could save a life. Emergency epinephrine kits are available in two self-administered delivery devices—a spring-loaded system (EpiPen) and a preloaded syringe (Ana-Kit). (See page 198 for further instructions.)

Food families
At one time, allergists recommended eliminating all foods from the same food family if one was known to cause allergies. In other words, if you had an allergy to peanut, you were supposed to avoid other legumes such as peas.

We now believe that although cross allergies are possible, they don't necessarily occur. Recent controlled double-blind studies have shown that cross-reactivity is very rare. Even people who have a severe life-threatening allergy to peanuts are unlikely to have reactions to other legumes. (Peanut is a legume, not a nut.) Diets that eliminate entire food families are therefore no longer considered necessary.

It is preferable to have as few foods as possible on the avoid list. That way, since only a few foods need to be eliminated, the diet will be easier to follow and there will be less chance of jeopardizing your nutritional balance.

Delaying food allergies in infants
If very young infants develop allergies, it is usually to cow's milk protein or cow's milk protein in formula, as this is the primary food during the first six months of life.

In these early months, infants are particularly susceptible to food allergies. They have what is sometimes described as a "leaky" or "open" digestive tract. The mucosal barrier that lines the intestine is immature; it sometimes allows proteins to enter the bloodstream before they are broken down. These whole proteins are more likely to stimulate the sensitization process and production of IgE antibodies.

As babies begin to eat solid foods, they may become sensitized to egg, soy and peanut. Allergy to wheat is less common, although some children cannot tolerate wheat because they have another disease, such as celiac disease.

Anything you can do to prevent food allergies in your infant or at least delay symptoms for several months is worthwhile. This prevention starts with your decision to breast-feed your baby. Exclusive breast-feeding (that means no other foods or formula) for four to six months is a good idea for all babies, and especially for babies who have a high risk of developing allergies.

Infants who develop allergies while being exclusively breast-fed do so because an allergen from something in the mother's diet—such as egg—is carried into her milk. When there is a strong likelihood that the infant is atopic, by restricting her own diet the nursing mother may be able to delay, but not necessarily prevent, her infant from developing allergies. Before doing this, the mother should discuss her diet with her doctor or a professional dietitian to ensure that she does not risk malnutrition.

If it is necessary to use a formula as a supplement or as a main feeding during the first four to six months, a non-allergic type is best. Soy formula is often used because it contains a different protein than milk, although 15 to 20 per cent of infants who are allergic to cow's milk protein will also react to soy as a separate reaction. The best advice is to talk to your physician before starting any formula and to do it cautiously, as this next case illustrates.

Baby Laura was exclusively breast-fed for the first five months of her life. Then, because of a family history of allergies, her mother used soy formula as the weaning milk. Immediately after finishing her first bottle, Laura started vomiting copiously; she became extremely pale and lost consciousness. Later, skin tests showed a positive response to cow's milk, egg, soy and peanut. Yet she'd never been fed any of these foods, except for the one bottle of soy formula. RAST analysis indicated she had IgE antibodies in her blood to these foods.

Based on these surprising findings, we concluded that Laura might be one of those rare infants who is highly allergic. Her only previous exposure to milk, egg, soy and peanut would have been through her mother's breast milk, but since the amounts would have been small, any sensitivity was not noticed until Laura had a full bottle of soy formula.

We want to emphasize that Laura's case is rare, but it does point out that serious allergic reactions in infants can be delayed by exclusive breast-feeding for the first four to six months.

Some research suggests that sensitization can even occur during pregnancy. When the risk of allergy is high, therefore, some doctors place mothers on special diets during the last three months of pregnancy. This is a controversial issue, and we aren't yet convinced of the value of these restrictions. Until there is more scientific evidence, we worry about jeopardizing the nutritional status of the mother and her fetus at such an important time.

Even though breast milk is highly nutritious, sometime around six months of age babies need additional foods for energy, for protein and for key nutrients, such as iron. The best way to minimize problems is to introduce new foods very slowly. A baby with a family history of allergies should be given only one new food a week, starting with one small spoonful. If there are no problems, you can increase the serving size over the next few days until your baby is receiving a full serving. By proceeding slowly, you'll have a chance to observe any initial or delayed adverse reactions.

Just because you notice some eczema, spitting up or diarrhea after the first introduction of a new food, don't jump to the conclusion that you have an allergic baby. There are any number of other reasons for temporary upsets. To be on the safe side, stop feeding the baby the new food for now but try it again in very small amounts a few weeks later, after all the symptoms have cleared. If you observe the same symptoms twice, discuss them with your doctor.

Initially all foods should be single ingredients. That means you start with plain cereals, such as rice cereal, rather than mixtures of several grains or cereal and fruit mixtures. Parents should develop a habit of reading ingredient labels in order to become more aware of the foods they are feeding their children.

Egg white or peanut butter should not be added to your infant's diet until close to the first birthday.

Children generally grow out of their allergies to milk or eggs, whereas peanut, nut and shellfish allergies are likely to continue for life.

Unusual food reactions
Allergists have documented a few unusual but interesting food allergen relationships.

The **fresh-fruit syndrome** occurs in individuals who are sensitive to trees, particularly birch. When these people eat certain fresh fruits or vegetables—such as apple, pear, cherry, carrot, potato or celery—they experience swelling and itching on their lips and inside their mouth. The reaction is uncomfortable, but not severe, and it never occurs with cooked fruits or vegetables. It would seem that the allergen is destroyed by heat.

A group of allergists in Italy have also found that many people with these fruit and vegetable allergies are also allergic to mugwort, a grass pollen. This is an example of an allergy cross-reaction.

A more serious unusual response is food-related **exercise-induced anaphylaxis**. If a person with this disease exercises within a few hours of eating a meal (fresh celery, fresh peaches and seafood are especially suspect), she develops hiving and respiratory symptoms that at times can be life-threatening.

A case recently reported in the medical literature is of a healthy nineteen-year-old male college athlete who, as part of his training for the wrestling team, ran daily. One day, his lunch was a shrimp salad. He'd eaten shellfish frequently in the past and had never had any allergy symptoms, but this time, three and one-half hours later, after a vigorous twenty-five-minute run, he noticed both hands felt numb, and his scalp, neck and arms were intensely itchy. He took a cold shower, followed by a warm shower, then noticed his face swelling; he had difficulty breathing and focusing. He felt as if he were going to pass out.

Fortunately, the team physician was close at hand and administered adrenaline. Within ten minutes, the signs and symptoms began to disappear.

Myths about food allergies

Although some children and adults do have food allergies, we're concerned that many people are limiting their diets unnecessarily. They mistakenly believe that food allergies are causing certain symptoms and decide to eliminate that food from their diet without proper diagnosis. Let's refute some common myths.

- **Colic is not a symptom of allergies.** Infantile colic, those unexplained, worrisome, prolonged episodes of irritability, fussiness or crying, is thought by some to be a sign of allergy to infant formula. But babies with colic rarely have elevated blood levels of IgE antibodies, suggestive of an allergic reaction. Although improvement sometimes occurs with a change in formula, other babies may be simply sucking too much air and need a nipple with a large hole.

  Colic also occurs in breast-fed babies. In that case, sometimes limiting milk in the mother's diet to one cup a day helps. If there is no change in a week, you'll have to look for other solutions. Extra holding, swaddling and rocking seem to be what some babies need.

  Fortunately, colic ends at about three to four months of age, and colicky babies grow and develop at normal rates. The main reason for treating the problem is to give parents some urgently needed rest and relief.
- **Mucus isn't a sign of milk allergy.** Many people feel that milk is a cause of excess mucus in the nose or lungs. They tend to relate nasal symptoms or worsening of their asthma with milk consumption. But there is no proven relationship between drinking milk and the production of mucus. Milk restriction is not warranted.

It is extremely rare for a food sensitivity to cause asthma, but when it does occur, it is obvious. The wheezing occurs immediately after the food is eaten.

- **Food allergies are not the cause of a host of vague symptoms.** Some adults blame food allergies for fatigue, depression, compulsive eating and drinking, memory loss and a host of other symptoms. But once again there is no scientific evidence of a cause-and-effect relationship.

- **Sugar does not cause hyperactivity.** Despite media reports that sugar, especially in large amounts, can cause hyperactivity in children, controlled research studies done in a double-blind fashion prove otherwise. Work at the University of Toronto has shown that sugar, in reasonable amounts, tends to have a calming effect on children. Other dietary factors may play a role in hyperactivity, but direct evidence is lacking at this time. Therefore we don't recommend aggressive dietary manipulation.

ADVERSE REACTIONS TO FOOD ADDITIVES

Many people are concerned that food additives may be causing problems such as wheezing, runny noses and skin rashes. Others believe that their children's hyperactivity is related to food additives, especially to food colouring agents.

A food additive is a substance that is not normally consumed by itself but is intentionally added to a food to enhance certain features of the food, such as texture, colour or flavour, or to prevent food spoilage.

There has been significant publicity surrounding these additives, to the point that some people advocate a complete ban on their use. Others believe many additives are essential in order to allow us to enjoy a wide variety of safe foods. Unfortunately, there has been, and continues to be, considerable confusion surrounding this subject.

Food additives can be divided into many different categories, depending on their function, but the ones commonly associated with adverse reactions fall into four general categories:

- food colouring agents
- preservatives
- flavour enhancers
- nutrient sweeteners

Although the Health Protection Branch of Health and Welfare Canada does study food additives in terms of the risk of their causing cancer and other diseases, it is impossible to predict which additives might cause allergy problems. This is because allergy problems occur only in certain individuals who, in turn, are sensitive to other things in their environment that don't bother most people. It is only after an additive has been in use for a long time that we might discover such relationships. For example, the discovery that sulphites could cause asthma attacks came to light because one patient cleverly reasoned that her attacks came on mainly when she drank a specific brand of white wine. The wine was eventually found to contain sulphites. Testing of other asthmatic patients eventually led to the discovery that 5 to 10 per cent of asthmatic patients are likely to have an asthma attack shortly after ingesting foods containing large amounts of sulphite preservative.

Despite many books and articles about food additives, controlled research studies are now showing that intolerance to food additives is much rarer than most people think. In one study in England, more than 18,000 people answered a

> **Adverse reactions to food additives are very rare.**

questionnaire about reactions to food or food additives. Fifteen per cent reported that they had symptoms caused by foods and 7 per cent thought that they could not tolerate certain food additives. More than 1,000 of these people were examined, but only 132 had recurring symptoms that justified further testing. Upon challenge testing with various additives and placebos, in a double-blind controlled fashion, as described on page 31, only three had reproducible symptoms. That suggests that the real prevalence of adverse reactions to food additives is less than 0.03 per cent.

One of our patients suspected that red food dye was causing her allergy problem. However, routine skin testing revealed an allergy to tomato. All the red foods that concerned the patient contained tomato paste. This is a clear example of why appropriate investigations are required in all cases.

Diagnosis

Despite symptoms resembling those associated with allergies—wheezing, hives, rhinitis—reactions to food additives are not mediated by an allergic mechanism. That is, they do not involve the IgE antibody as discussed in Chapter 1. This means that we cannot use skin or blood tests to evaluate adverse reactions to additives, as we do with allergies to specific foods, such as milk and egg. This is one situation where we do use a form of elimination diet. We ask the patient to avoid all the foods that contain the suspect additive for at least ten to fourteen days to see if the symptoms disappear. Since additives are found in so many foods, we ask a dietitian to help plan these diets. Sometimes we try to eliminate just one particular food additive; other times we eliminate several additives. In cases that are extremely severe or puzzling, we can use a very restricted diet in which the patient drinks only certain commercial preparations containing alternative non-allergic nutrient sources.

If the patient improves on the diet, we then give her a challenge dose of the suspect additive. This must be done in a setting, such as the doctor's office or hospital emergency room, where appropriate treatment of any reactions can be easily performed. Challenge testing is done either openly—that is the patient knows what she is receiving— or double blind. In some cases where the cause is more evident, we proceed directly to challenging the patient with the suspect additive without bothering with the elimination diet.

Food colouring agents

Since children tend to be especially fond of brightly coloured foods, food dyes are often blamed for children's health problems. In Canada, the six major dyes used in foods are Tartrazine, Sunset Yellow FCF, Amaranth, Erythrosine, Brilliant Blue FCF and Indigotine. There are others such as Fast Green FCF, Allura Red and Ponceau 5X that are used less often.

Tartrazine is the major food dye implicated in adverse reactions. It appears in cake and icing mixes, cheese-flavoured snacks, puddings, pie fillings and gelatin desserts, ice creams and sherbets, drink mixes and soft drinks and medications. It is often blamed for nasal stuffiness, asthma and hives. The other dyes have rarely been associated with problems.

One research study investigating the relationship between Tartrazine and asthma showed the importance of double-blind testing. When forty-five people with severe asthma were tested with foods they knew contained Tartrazine, seven reacted. When these same patients were tested with foods that disguised the Tartrazine (a double-blind challenge), none developed asthma. This and other studies now suggest that the frequency of Tartrazine allergy has been overemphasized.

An interesting aspect of Tartrazine reactions is that some reported cases have been in people who are also sensitive to Aspirin, but scientists have not been able to discover a chemical explanation for this cross-reactivity. At the Scripps Clinic in La Jolla, California, the doctors have been performing double-blind challenges with Tartrazine on all Aspirin-sensitive asthmatic patients. After more than 165 such challenges, they have yet to find one person with a positive response to Tartrazine.

In 1973, Dr. Benjamin Feingold took concerns about Tartrazine one step further. He wrote a popular book that blamed hyperactivity, behaviour problems and learning disabilities in children on Tartrazine, other food colouring agents such as Amaranth, and natural salicylates in foods. Parents who were anxiously seeking explanations for their children's difficult behaviour embraced Feingold's theory and placed their children on a diet that restricted all foods containing artificial colours and flavours, and natural salicylates. Feingold claimed that 50 per cent of hyperactive children improved with this diet. Many parents also believed it worked.

Since that time, many double-blind controlled studies have failed to show a relationship between diet and behaviour in school. Some children under five years of age may have been helped by such a diet, but certainly not as many as claimed by Feingold.

In addition, his diet is not easy to use. It requires significant additional food preparation and extensive training from a dietitian. The Feingold diet has been around for almost twenty years, and the problem is far from being cured. We have little confidence in it and do not recommend it.

Hyperactivity is similar to asthma in complexity. With asthma, you cannot hope to alleviate the problem by singling out one culprit and removing it from your environment. A comprehensive program of asthma management involves minimizing many environmental contacts and using medication. No doubt effective treatment of hyperactivity, when developed, will also be multifaceted.

We are concerned that many teachers believe that certain foods, usually labelled "junk foods," cause behavioural problems in the classroom. Faced with inattentive or unruly students, teachers often inappropriately advise parents to seek dietary counselling. Behavioural problems are very complex and must be examined thoroughly.

Preservatives
For six centuries, sulphites have prevented spoilage and colour change in foods. But in about 5 per cent of asthmatics, sulphites can precipitate symptoms. Symptoms

can range from mild wheezing to life-threatening asthmatic episodes. These reactions can come on within twenty to thirty minutes of eating a particular food, and this is how one can begin to suspect they are causing the problem.

Sulphite agents—including sodium sulphite, sulphur dioxide, sodium and potassium bisulphites—prevent browning of potatoes, lettuce and other salad ingredients, sanitize and inhibit the growth of undesirable microorganisms during the making of wine and beer, and protect scallops and shrimps from spoilage. A wide variety of processed foods—from soups and jams, to juices, to sausage meats, to dried fruits, to frozen pies and pastries—may contain sulphites. On frozen or canned foods, the sulphite ingredients are listed on the label.

In the past, restaurants in Canada often used sulphite solutions to keep the ingredients on their salad bars looking fresher longer. A normal daily intake of sulphites would be only ten milligrams in food prepared at home but one restaurant meal might have contained as much as 100 to 400 milligrams of sulphite preservative. There is now a law in Canada banning the use of sulphites on fruits and vegetables sold or served raw to consumers, but you can't be 100 per cent sure. Packaged chopped raw vegetables labelled preservative-free may have been washed in water containing sulphite. Thus restaurant owners can't be absolutely sure that the fruits or vegetables they're buying from Mexico, Arizona or California are sulphite free. Imported grapes, for example, might have sulphite on them.

People with sulphite sensitivity must be very cautious, especially when eating out. At home, they are safest when buying locally grown produce and rinsing it well.

Test strips are sold that are supposed to detect the presence of sulphite compounds in foods, but they can't be relied upon to be consistently accurate. The strips may not test low enough to be accurate for the person with a high degree of sensitivity; also, the results can be affected by acid in foods such as fruit and salad dressings. Even when the strip registers negative, the food may not be safe to eat.

Although foods are the major source of sulphite compounds, they aren't the only one. Studies show that levels of sulphur dioxide from air pollution in some areas may be sufficient to cause wheezing in highly sensitized people, especially if exercise follows exposure.

Drugs, even some used to treat asthma, also contain sulphite compounds as preservatives and antioxidants. Fortunately, the sulphite compounds have been removed from many drugs and reduced in others to a low concentration so as not to be a significant problem. Occasionally, a person will have an asthma attack after taking a medication. In such a case, the possibility of sulphite contamination should be considered.

Butylated hydroxyanisole (BHA) and butylated hydroxytoluene (BHT) are commonly used as antioxidants in breakfast cereals and other grain products to maintain crispness and in oils to prevent rancidity. Despite some concerns, there have been no well-documented reports of hypersensitivity to these agents when consumed in the amounts permitted in foods. Although some sources suggest using large doses of BHT as an anti-aging, anti-cancer or anti-herpes agent, excessive doses of BHT could be toxic.

Sodium benzoate and benzoic acid are effective anti-microbial preservatives used in foods such as cereals, cakes and instant potatoes. Benzoic acid also occurs naturally in many foods such as cranberries, raspberries, prunes, tea, cinnamon, cloves and anise.

Feingold includes benzoate in his list of food ingredients that may cause behavioural problems (see page 129), but that claim has not been substantiated.

Some studies have shown that benzoates may cause hives or swelling, but these reactions occurred more often when the preservatives were used in drugs rather than in foods. A very small number of patients in a few studies did wheeze after using these compounds in foods, but the studies indicated that very few people are sensitive to these preservatives.

Some allergists suspect that cross-reactivity between benzoates, BHT, BHA and Aspirin do occur, but the studies to date have yielded varying results.

Nitrates are used in cured meats—ham, salami and weiners—to prevent deadly botulism. Although it has not been proven that they cause hypersensitivity reactions, some people find they do provoke headaches similar to migraine headaches, or what we commonly call "the hot dog headache."

Flavour enhancers

The flavour enhancer monosodium glutamate (MSG) is one of the most widely used food additives. It is added to many canned and packaged soups, bouillon cubes, soy sauce, salad dressings, frozen dinners and appetizers. The average daily intake is less than one gram, but a Chinese meal may contain five to ten grams. Hence, the characteristic symptoms that occur following ingestion of large amounts of MSG—numbness at the back of the neck radiating to both arms, general weakness, heart palpitations, dizziness, chest pain, abdominal cramps, nausea, vomiting and headaches—have been dubbed the "Chinese Restaurant Syndrome." These symptoms may occur twenty to thirty minutes after eating. As a separate reaction, asthma can begin one to two hours after a meal or, in some patients, twelve to fourteen hours after the meal. These attacks can vary from mild to life threatening.

Fortunately, publicity has alerted many food manufacturers to this problem, and now you will see labels on foods showing that they no longer contain MSG. When eating in restaurants, you are not able to determine all the ingredients. The chef may not even realize that the soy sauce he uses contains MSG, for example. The Canadian Restaurant and Foodservice Association is well aware of this problem and is encouraging education of food-service workers.

Some allergy groups are lobbying to have food ingredient information printed on menus. But restaurants often must substitute ingredients when they have a peak demand for a certain dish. Although their normal supplier might send MSG-free or sulphite-free ingredients, a last-minute substitute might contain these or other additives. That's why it is better to ask about today's ingredients from a staff member who is knowledgeable rather than rely on possibly out-dated information printed on a menu.

Aspartame is a low-calorie sweetener marketed under the brand name of NutraSweet. It is used in carbonated beverages, fruit juices, gums, frozen desserts, breath mints, iced tea, vitamins and cereals. A few reports have surfaced describing reactions such as hives or swelling that have occurred a few hours after its ingestion, but the number of patients so affected is very small. Recently, allergists in Bethesda, Maryland, advertised extensively for thirty-two months to find people who might have a hypersensitivity to aspartame. In that time they found no one who, in a double-blind challenge, had clearly reproducible adverse reactions to aspartame. Thus, controlled studies have failed to reveal any adverse reactions to aspartame, including headaches (see page 31).

Treatment

Appropriate treatment consists of avoiding the particular additive associated with the problem. But to avoid food additives, one must know which foods contain them. Although packaged foods have ingredient listings on the label, many foods are not packaged and labelled. As well, smaller food manufacturers may not be meticulous about including sub-ingredients on the label. For example, an ingredient label may list soy sauce but not the MSG in the soy sauce. Gradually, legislation is changing to improve consumer information, but in the meantime patient advocacy groups, along with concerned physicians, need to lobby more strongly for changes.

Eating out can be particularly difficult, as described above, but often the problem is closer to home. When your neighbour bakes a cake for her son's birthday party, she may not be aware that some of the ingredients she is using could be dangerous for your child.

Because of the distinct possibility of accidental ingestion, any person or the parents of a child who has previously had a severe reaction to a food additive must always be prepared by carrying an injectable form of adrenaline, an Ana-Kit or EpiPen. These have an immediate beneficial effect, but are used only for severe, life-threatening reactions. After an adrenaline injection, the person should be taken to the emergency department of the nearest hospital for evaluation and further treatment.

For milder reactions, use an antihistamine tablet (or liquid for children). Specific brands are best recommended by your physician.

As with foods, food additives are not responsible for allergic reactions as often as most people think. Each individual has their own internal make-up and responds to many things in the environment, not just foods. This is why it is important to seek medical help when problems occur so that any diseases, especially those that are not obvious to the patient, can be ruled out. Whenever food additives are suspect, seek help from allergists experienced in this area in order to arrange for proper elimination diets and for challenge tests.

CHAPTER SEVEN

Allergic Skin Diseases

Most people have had a skin rash that went away on its own before the cause was found. Persistent rashes, however, can be ugly, embarrassing, itchy and uncomfortable. Children often scratch rashes to the point that they become infected.

Allergists commonly treat eczema (atopic dermatitis), in which the skin is red and very itchy, with either dry, flaky patches or wet, weepy areas, and hives (urticaria), which is characterized by white, raised areas (wheals) surrounded by redness. Sometimes the hives look like mosquito bites; sometimes they appear as large welts. They are usually intensely itchy.

Eczema

Although the exact cause of eczema is unknown, we do know that about 80 per cent of children with eczema have allergies. Yet allergies do not cause the eczema. There is a tendency to inherit eczema and in the presence of allergy inflammation there is a worsening of the eczema.

The human skin

Normal, healthy skin is an essential protective barrier against the outside world. Although most people think of skin as a thin covering, it is the largest organ in the human body.

Your skin has three layers: a thin outer protective, epidermis layer; a middle, dermis layer where the blood vessels, nerves, sweat glands and hair roots are located; and an inner, subcutaneous layer consisting mainly of insulating fat cells.

It's the epidermis and dermis layers that have the most significance to allergists. The epidermis cells are continually being replaced. Old cells become flatter and tougher as they age. Eventually they die and are sloughed off. Each day we shed up to one gram of dead cells into our bath, clothes and bedding. It's these dead cells that provide ready food for dust mites, a common source of allergen (see Chapter 2).

The mast cells, which play such an important role in allergies, are in the dermis layer. When they release histamine and other mediators into the skin, you develop inflammation—redness, swelling and itching associated with eczema and hives.

By now, you'll realize that the allergic immune response is complicated, but our understanding of this response and how it creates inflammation has increased enormously in the last few years. We've learned that the allergic immune response is more than positive skin tests and more than IgE antibodies on mast cells. It also includes a series of immune cells that respond to allergens. Inflammation in the skin of patients with eczema is likely due to this cellular activity. This is similar to the cellular changes that occur in the lungs of a person with asthma.

There is still much controversy over the relationship between allergy and skin rashes. Many parents are convinced their child's rash is caused by an allergy to a food, such as milk, but in fact the relationship between allergy and eczema is still not well understood.

We believe that in the next few years, a better understanding of this eczema-allergy relationship will emerge as we discover more about how the allergic immune response works to create inflammation. In the meantime, our limited understanding of inflammation provides a rationale for the ways we manage eczema.

About 3 per cent of infants and young children develop eczema at some time, and this can be a very worrisome problem for parents. The itchy, weepy rashes can make your baby irritable and sleepless, and if your child scratches the rash, it could become infected. Fortunately, eczema tends to improve with age; it is less common in older children and adults.

In babies, eczema usually appears as a weepy, scaly rash on the cheeks, scalp, neck, backs of the arms, fronts of the legs or trunk. You may even notice your baby rubbing his or her face on a pillow or cot side in an attempt to relieve the itching. In older infants and toddlers, eczema is usually localized in skin folds, behind the knees, inside the elbows, at the wrists and ankles and at the side of the neck. In older children and adults, eczema on hands and feet and around the nipples and lips is common.

During the first two years of life, eczema is more common in those infants who have allergies—that is, who have IgE antibodies. As we discussed in Chapter 6, infant allergies are usually to food proteins—especially milk, eggs, peanut butter, nuts and fish. When an infant has severe eczema, it is worth investigating the possibility of food allergies.

We do want to stress, however, that food allergy alone is not as common a cause of eczema as many people think. Even if there is a positive skin test to a food, it does not always mean that a food allergy is the cause of the eczema. Proving the relationship may require a food challenge test supervised by your doctor. Certainly we never recommend very restrictive diets in the treatment of eczema.

> **The presence of a positive skin test to a food does not prove the food is causing the eczema.**

As we discussed in Chapter 6, it is typical for young children to outgrow food allergies. Children who have had significant eczema in infancy often switch to a sensitivity to airborne allergens at about age two or three and the eczema persists. At this time, it is not clear whether airborne allergens play a role in aggravating eczema. We do know that about half the children with atopic eczema also have asthma, while 60 per cent of children with troublesome asthma experience eczema at some time.

As happens with asthma, the inflammation occurring with eczema can be aggravated by other factors as well as allergies. Patients need to consider many other things, such as contact irritation from rough clothing, soaps and detergents. Even excessive moisture from perspiration and climate extremes—both cold, dry air and hot, humid weather—may aggravate eczema. The dust mite, which breeds in your mattress and carpeting, has also been shown to be a factor in eczema. Before jumping to the conclusion that eczema is a sign that you are allergic to one or many foods, consider all the possible aggravating factors.

Treatment of eczema

Although we cannot cure eczema, we can effectively control it with medications that decrease the inflammation in the skin, and with non-specific lotions and creams designed to improve the skin's health.

Itching as a result of the inflammation in the skin starts a vicious cycle. You scratch; that leads to more eczema rash; the rash is itchy; and the cycle repeats itself. The best medications for controlling this cycle are the topical steroids, which are anti-inflammatory—that is, they reduce inflammation and swelling. We also use oral antihistamine medications, which block the action of histamine, a mediator that causes the itching.

For mild eczema, the steroid most commonly used is hydrocortisone in an ointment or cream form. If the inflammation is more severe, we will prescribe more potent steroids, such as betamethasone. Only the milder forms of medication should be used on the face.

With eczema, the skin tends to be dry, so we suggest that you lubricate your skin with moisturizing creams and after-bath oils and use only non-irritating soaps. When buying soaps, look for the word "hypoallergenic" on the label. It means the product is not as likely to cause allergies—but you can never be sure, as individual responses vary.

Ways to reduce eczema problems

- When possible, keep the temperature of your house (or at least the bedrooms) at 20°C and the humidity between 25 and 40 per cent. (See Chapter 5 for suggestions on temperature and humidity control.)
- Protect your skin from cold weather with creams and emollients before going outside and at bedtime.
- Keep your fingernails short and clean so there is less chance of tearing and infecting the skin. Children may have to wear gloves at night to prevent scratching.
- Wear cotton; it is much less likely to irritate the skin than wool, silk, polyester or nylon.
- Use only small amounts of mild soaps, as recommended by your physician, for bathing and washing clothes. Rinse thoroughly. Many detergents and perfumed soaps irritate the skin.
- Bath daily, but keep your soaking time to 5 to 10 minutes. Apply a non-allergenic moisturizer immediately afterward to protect the skin from becoming too dry.

If scratching has led to a secondary skin infection, we will also prescribe a course of antibiotics—to be taken either orally or applied to the skin.

Even if you do follow all your doctor's instructions carefully, there may be times when the eczema flares up for no apparent reason. Using a steroid ointment at these times will help to relieve the inflammation. These are relatively safe medications—as safe as the inhaled forms of steroid that we use in the treatment of asthma. However, overuse of any medication is dangerous. Therefore be sure your doctor knows how frequently you are using the ointments so he or she can monitor your response.

In addition, in the box on page 144, we've suggested a few measures you can take to help yourself or your child feel more comfortable.

Contact dermatitis

Contact dermatitis, a type of skin disease, can occur when an irritating substance comes in direct contact with the skin. The skin becomes itchy and red, and blisters and crusts can form. Probably the best known example is the reaction to poison ivy, but resins from oak and sumac leaves often cause dermatitis in sensitive individuals. With a bit of simple sleuthing, you will probably be able to find the cause and eliminate it. The rash usually appears within twenty-four to forty-eight hours after contact with the offending substance, so think about any new products you just started using. Also, consider new supplies of old favourites, as sometimes manufacturers change the formulation of their products without stating it on the label. The box that follows can help you in your search.

If the cause isn't obvious, your allergist or dermatologist can do skin patch tests (see Chapter 2). Until your skin has healed, avoid excessive wetting, protect against cuts and grazes and use non-perfumed moisturizing creams and ointments to keep your skin from chapping.

Common causes of contact dermatitis

- soap, cleansing cream, bubble bath and detergent
- shampoo, conditioner, mousse, hairspray
- shaving cream and after-shave lotion
- perfume, cosmetic, lipstick, eye shadow, mascara, nail varnish
- toothpaste, mouthwash, gargling rinse
- deodorant, depilatory
- contraceptive cream or jelly, diaphragms, condoms, douche additives, vaginal medication, menstrual pads, tampons
- athlete's foot remedies, foot powder
- dye or perfume in toilet paper
- nickel in earring studs and other jewellery, lipstick cases, jean studs, button shanks and zippers, coins and key chains in your pocket
- plastic and rubber in garment waistbands, girdles and socks, stereo headphones, telephone receivers
- agents used to tan leather for clothing, gloves, shoes, slippers, boots

---

Hives

When a patient comes to see us about hives, we try to determine whether his rash was acute, that is, one that came on suddenly and lasted for just a few minutes or days; whether it is chronic, persisting for six weeks or more—even years; or recurrent (coming and going). This helps us determine the possible causes.

The acute form of hives is most often associated with an allergic response to a food or drug. Hives may even occur during an infection, such as a cold. They can also be part of the allergic response to an insect sting, as will be discussed in Chapter 9. Your history and skin testing can help us discover possible causes. If the food is something that you eat only occasionally, the hives may be recurrent.

Hives that are a result of an allergic reaction generally respond readily to antihistamines and don't return if you avoid the allergen.

Ten-month-old Ivan developed an acute case of hives within minutes of tasting eggs for the first time. He'd had mild eczema in the past, but didn't seem to be having any difficulty tolerating cow's milk and wheat. Our skin tests showed that Ivan was indeed allergic to eggs, and we removed them from his diet. A course of antihistamines cleared his hives.

Every six months, we repeated the skin test. Eventually, when the tests yielded negative results we gave Ivan a very little egg while he was in our office. (See the description of challenge testing on page 30.) At this point, he was able to tolerate egg and could now have it regularly in his diet.

Byron was brought to our offices when he was two years old. He'd had many ear infections in the past, which were usually treated with penicillin. Now he had generalized hives that had begun when he was on penicillin. We administered a skin test and found that Byron was allergic to penicillin, but to none of the other substances we tried. The hives were cleared up with antihistamines, and we advised Byron's parents to ensure he was never given penicillin again, as the next reaction could be more severe. As a warning sign for other doctors who might be treating Byron in an emergency, we suggested that he wear a Medic-Alert bracelet. (See page 159.)

There is a type of swelling—called **angioedema**—that occurs in the deeper layers of the skin in various and widespread parts of the body. It often accompanies the formation of hives or may occur by itself. With angioedema, the face, mouth and lips may become so swollen that the person's appearance is totally changed. If the swelling involves the throat and vocal cords, the person may have difficulty breathing and death could result if not immediately treated. In the previous chapter, we told you about Larry, a young boy who was allergic to peanut and who developed angioedema after eating a peanut butter cookie.

There is also a rare form of angioedema that is not accompanied by hives and itching and is not associated with allergies. Rather, it is an inherited disorder for which there is as yet no known cure, but we are able to reduce the swelling and frequency of attacks with special medication.

Non-allergic hives

Chronic or recurrent hives, that is, hives that last for more than six weeks or recur in crops weeks or months later, are usually caused by something other than allergies. Other things besides IgE antibodies can begin the sequence of reactions that ultimately results in inflammation. Some of these are:

- infectious diseases, such as infectious hepatitis or mononucleosis, fungus or parasite infections and intestinal worms
- physical pressure—tight clothing, carrying heavy weights or excessive rubbing of the skin

- sunlight
- cold temperatures—sometimes the hives appear when the skin is warmed, after exposure to cold
- insect bites—mosquitos, bedbugs and fleas (see Chapter 9)
- x-ray dyes and certain drugs, such as Aspirin, penicillin and steroids (Note: Drugs can cause both allergic hives and non-allergic hives. See Chapter 8.)

Chuck's hives began in October and persisted for about six months before his mother brought him to our office. This seven-year-old also had mild symptoms of hay fever and eczema, and our skin testing showed he was allergic to dust and dust mites. We were able to prove, however, that the hives were due not to allergy but to a reaction to cold. We held an ice cube over his arm for about five minutes and then rewarmed the skin. Immediately, a hive in the shape of the ice cube appeared. Treatment consisted of antihistamine medication on a regular basis until the hive no longer occurred when the ice was applied to his skin. Extra care was needed in covering Chuck's skin when dressing for the outdoors. No treatment was necessary over the summer months. The next winter, there was some recurrence of the hives, but the episodes were not nearly as severe.

Many times we never do discover what initially caused the hives, but we are able to shut down the process that leads to the hiving by using many of the same drugs we use for allergies—that is, antihistamine and the anti-inflammatory medications, such as prednisone. Avoidance is not part of the management strategy.

Ten-year-old Cathy first developed chronic hives after an upper respiratory infection. Treatment with antihistamine

*provided some relief, but the hives did not disappear entirely.
We tested her for allergies and found none. Neither could we
find any possible diseases. We know her hives are not a result
of sunlight, cold or pressure, but we are able to raise a welt by
stroking her skin. Thus, there is little we can do at this time
to prevent the hives, but we can control their severity with
antihistamines.*

Very rarely, hives indicate an underlying disease, such as
cancer or some immune disorder. For example, with auto-
immune thyroiditis, there are hives associated with the
thyroid disorder. There are diagnostic procedures that
can rule out these possibilities.

A number of women who have never before had
allergy problems develop hives during pregnancy. We
even have a name for the condition—**pregnancy urticaria**. This isn't a sign of any serious or long-term problem,
unless the hives are accompanied by extensive swelling.
To relieve irritation or itching, it is safe to use topical
antihistamines.

What can you do?

It's not necessary to seek medical help for occasional
minor bouts of hives, as they will probably disappear on
their own. If hives persist for several days, or recur, think
carefully about all possible triggers. Also, consider your
general health. Have you had a recent cold or infection?
Are there other recurring allergy symptoms? See your
doctor and be sure to give him or her all this information.

As treatment, your doctor will probably start you on
one of the antihistamine medications. He or she may
have to try different products until he or she finds the one

that works best for you. Be patient; it will take a few days of treatment to achieve results.

As long as the hives are present, avoid exposure to irritants such as wool clothing, detergents, perfumes and soaps. Do not take any ASA-containing medications, such as Aspirin.

For acute hives with extensive swelling and breathing difficulties, get to a doctor or emergency department of a hospital immediately. You may need an adrenaline injection. As we discuss in Chapters 6 and 9, **people who are known to develop angioedema as a result of a severe reaction to peanut or insect stings should carry an adrenaline kit (EpiPen or Ana-Kit) with them at all times.**

CHAPTER EIGHT

Reactions to Drugs and Vaccines

When patients first learn that the rash, itchy hives, swelling or upset stomach they had was an adverse reaction to a drug, they are upset—even angry. "Why didn't my doctor warn me?"

If their reaction is to an over-the-counter drug such as Aspirin, a cold remedy or skin cream, they ask, "Why is this drug sold without a prescription?" or "Why wasn't there a warning on the label?"

When one member of a family has a serious drug reaction, the others ask, "Can you test me to see if I'm also allergic?" Sometimes that's possible, but as we'll explain, it often isn't.

ADVERSE REACTIONS TO DRUGS

The use of medications of any sort, even those applied to the skin, is not without risk, but only a very small percentage of adverse reactions to drugs are true allergies. The majority of adverse reactions, about 80 per cent, are predictable problems such as overdose and side effects. Often your doctor will warn you about such possible side effects when giving you a prescription.

Predictable adverse reactions to drugs

> If young children are around, keep all drugs, even iron supplements, stored in locked cupboards. Never refer to drugs as candy.

Drug toxicity results from taking too much of a drug—an overdose—either accidentally or deliberately. Taking the exact amount of a prescribed drug is important; more is not better.

Drug side effects are unpleasant but sometimes unavoidable actions of the drug. The antibiotic erythromycin can cause abdominal cramps, nausea, vomiting and diarrhea. Antihistamines used in treating allergic disorders may cause drowsiness. With some drugs, lowering the dose or altering the time you take the drug (before bed or with meals) may help. If the side effects are severe, the drug will have to be discontinued.

Secondary drug effects are indirect consequences unrelated to the drug's primary action. After repeated or prolonged use of certain antibiotics, bacteria may flourish in your intestinal tract, producing diarrhea. Similarly, steroid inhalers may cause an overgrowth of certain fungi in the mouth.

Drug interactions can occur when two drugs are taken together and one interferes with the absorption or effectiveness of the other. This is why it is important to inform your doctor of all medications you are using, even over-the-counter preparations such as laxatives, vitamins, pain relievers, etc. Drugs that are quite safe when taken by themselves may create problems when taken in combination with other drugs.

When drugs are taken with foods, they may also have their effectiveness altered. Always check with your doctor or pharmacist as to how and when the drug should be taken.

None of these predictable reactions are allergic conditions. Thus, although you may have to discontinue taking the medication this time, it is quite unlikely that the reactions would recur if the drug were needed again at a later date.

Unpredictable drug reactions

Less than 20 per cent of drug reactions are unpredictable but some of these can be very serious. Unpredictable reactions occur because your individual body chemistry is slightly different than the norm. An inherited trait may not come to light until you have a reaction. Sometimes a tendency to react to a certain drug runs in a family. Knowledge of your family medical history can then serve as a warning that you may have difficulties with certain drugs.

Drug intolerance problems often resemble overdose symptoms, but they occur in certain patients taking average doses of the drug. An example is ringing in the ears after taking ASA-containing medication, such as Aspirin. This is a common side effect from a large dose, but some people experience it even when taking just a normal amount. There are no blood tests to detect these intolerances.

Drug idiosyncrasy is an inherited inability to handle certain drugs in any dose. Some members of African and

Mediterranean ethnic groups lack a certain enzyme in their red blood cells that makes them unable to tolerate medications such as sulpha and Aspirin, as well as many over-the-counter cold remedies. This particular defect can be detected with a blood test.

Allergic reactions are those in which an immune mechanism of antibodies, T lymphocytes and mediators is involved. In this case the drug, or a part of the drug, is the antigen. Probably the best-known drug allergy is to penicillin, but some people are allergic to other antibiotics, as well as a host of other drugs.

The symptoms of drug allergies, such as hives or swelling, are similar to those normally associated with other allergic reactions we've discussed in this book. They occur in only a minority of patients using the drug and do not resemble the usual side effects of the drug.

> **Drug allergies are rarely inherited. Even though you may have allergic diseases such as asthma, hay fever, eczema or food allergies, it doesn't mean you are more prone to drug allergies and vice versa.**

The first time you have an allergic reaction to a drug it will probably occur after you've been taking the drug for a week or so. That's because you must become sensitized by exposure to the drug. Occasionally, people don't realize they've been exposed to a particular drug, as in the example of penicillin in cow's milk (see page 13). Once sensitized, the reaction can occur within minutes to hours of taking even very tiny doses of the drug. This reaction may be reproduced each time you take the drug.

Because you must be sensitized to a drug before you respond to conventional allergy tests, it's very difficult to predict who will have drug allergies. Compared with other allergies, the inherited tendency isn't as strong. In other words, just because your parents have drug allergies, don't assume you have them.

Diagnosing drug allergies

Although some drugs do have characteristic responses that can help the doctor identify the culprit drug, we stress that any drug can produce any type of allergic response. To complicate matters, certain diseases cause the same reactions. For example, rashes from viral infections, such as colds, are very similar to rashes caused by various antibiotics.

In general, we suspect a reaction is due to a drug allergy when we have no other adequate explanation for the reaction; the reaction is different from the usual course of the illness; the timing is appropriate; the reaction is suggestive of something we would normally see when taking the drug; the reaction subsides within a few days of stopping the drug. That's why it is important to keep lists of medicines you have taken, including over-the-counter medications, and a diary of any abnormal drug reactions in the past.

To investigate a drug allergy after it has occurred once, we can sometimes use the allergy skin tests (prick and intradermal) or the RAST blood analysis described in Chapter 2.

If a patient has a history suggestive of drug allergies, and skin testing as well as blood tests are negative or, more likely, not available, then giving the patient the drug the next time he is ill is the only way left to establish an allergy.

This **provocative testing** is hazardous. It should be

done only if the drug in question is the only option for treating a particular illness and the benefit of taking the drug is greater than the risks involved. The test must be performed in the hospital with emergency equipment close at hand. A very weak solution of the drug in question is first tested on the skin by the prick test and then the intradermal technique. If that goes well, the intradermal testing is repeated at fifteen-minute intervals, with the drug dose increased tenfold each time until the dose reaches full strength. If there has been no reaction, the drug is given by the desired route, perhaps by mouth, once again starting with a very small dose and increasing gradually to the normal dose. Provocative testing must be done immediately before treatment is given, not weeks or months earlier.

Allergic reactions to non-prescription drugs

> **Treat over-the-counter drugs as seriously as prescription drugs. Read labels carefully.**

It's so easy to buy ASA-containing pain relievers, vitamins and skin creams without prescription that we tend to forget they're drugs. Most people tolerate them well, but in the susceptible person any one of them could cause an allergic reaction such as hives, swelling, breathing difficulties, vomiting or diarrhea. Some people who have asthma find that ASA-containing pain relievers or other arthritic medications aggravate their condition and may precipitate an asthma attack. When discussing disease symptoms with your doctor, be sure to mention any cold remedies, laxatives, sedatives, tonics, douches, suppositories and ointments you've been using.

As a marketing ploy, manufacturers sometimes imply

that medications made with all natural ingredients are safer. But natural compounds are just as likely to cause allergic reactions. Natural is not necessarily better. In fact, some herbal remedies, including herbal vitamins, can be very toxic in large doses.

Allergic reactions to drug additives

The amount of an active ingredient in most medicines is very small and rarely are these ingredients palatable, so drug manufacturers add fillers and colouring and fla-vouring agents. The extra ingredients can occasionally precipitate an adverse reaction, although, as with food additives, recent research indicates that such reactions aren't as common as once thought. One additive recently associated with adverse reactions is the preservative so-dium metabisulphite, used in some asthma medications. It causes severe wheezing in 5 to 10 per cent of asthmat-ics. Now that this is known, the preservative is being replaced in most such preparations.

Skin testing is not an appropriate means of investigat-ing reactions to additives, as they usually do not cause problems via the IgE pathway. Ingesting or inhaling these substances under controlled conditions in a hospital or doctor's office is the only testing means available, but it is time-consuming and cumbersome and, therefore, is done only in select cases.

Allergic reactions to antibiotics

The most common drug allergy we see is to **penicillin**, which affects up to 10 per cent of the population. Reac-tions to penicillin can range from mild rashes to life-threatening collapse. In the past, we stopped using penicillin any time a patient developed a rash and la-belled the person allergic to penicillin. Now that we are able to test for penicillin allergy, we find that close to 90 per cent of patients who have had a rash in the past while on penicillin can actually use the antibiotic safely. The rashes were likely from the infection, not the drug.

> *Darlene is a ten-year-old girl sent to our clinic for assessment of a possible penicillin allergy. When she was four years old, she'd been given amoxicillin, a form of penicillin, for an ear infection. During the treatment, she developed a rash and some swelling of her lips and eyelids. The amoxicillin was stopped and Darlene was labelled as allergic to penicillin. For subsequent infections, her doctor prescribed alternative drugs, such as erythromycin or sulpha medications. When we tested Darlene for penicillin allergy, using the prick and intradermal skin tests, the results were negative. We gave her a challenge dose of penicillin by mouth while she was in our offices, where we could immediately treat any adverse reaction. Darlene did not have a reaction and subsequently was able to tolerate a full course of penicillin.*

Penicillin is the only drug allergy we can assess with some accuracy by skin testing. It is 100 per cent effective at predicting life-threatening (or anaphylactic) reactions and can relieve many concerns about penicillin allergy. If testing shows you are allergic to penicillin, then you have a 50 to 70 per cent chance of having a life-threatening reaction (that is, anaphylaxis) if penicillin is given to you again.

There are other non-allergic reactions that can occur with penicillin. Although some of these can be severe, they are not life-threatening. Skin testing cannot predict whether these types of problems will occur; hence, if penicillin is needed and the skin tests are negative, we must weigh the benefits versus the risks.

Patients who are allergic to penicillin must also avoid all penicillin medications—drugs such as ampicillin, amoxicillin, Pondocillin, Penbritin and Clavulin, to name a few. In addition, there is a 5 to 10 per cent chance that you will also react to medications from the other group of antibiotics, the cephalosporin family (see below).

If you must have penicillin but are allergic to it, a process called desensitization can be used. The technique is similar to that previously described as provocative testing, except even smaller doses are given initially and in a slower fashion. It also must be done in hospital; the procedure is effective only at the time and would need to be repeated each time penicillin is needed.

> If you are allergic to penicillin, wear a Medic-Alert bracelet or carry a wallet card to prevent doctors from administering penicillin should you be ill or seriously injured and cannot speak for yourself. Contact the Canadian Medic-Alert Foundation, P.O. Box 9800, Station A, Don Mills, Ontario, M3C 2T9, (416) 696-0267

Allergies to drugs in the **cephalosporin** family can also be very severe. These drugs include Keflex and Ceclor. Typical symptoms are skin rashes such as hives; swelling of the face, eyelids or lips; puffiness of the hands and feet; and arthritis or pain in the joints. **Serum sickness** is a term used to describe this complex of symptoms when they occur together following drug treatment. It can be very debilitating.

As mentioned above, people who are allergic to penicillin often have a cross-reaction with Ceclor. Any person

Anyone who has a known allergy to penicillin should not be given cephalosporin drugs.

with a known penicillin allergy should not be given any cephalosporin medications. Testing for cephalosporin allergy is not as common as testing for penicillin allergy, as it is neither effective nor reliable.

Chuck had a reaction to a course of penicillin given when he was two years old. At that time, he developed a rash, swelling and breathing difficulties. Because of this suspected penicillin allergy, his doctor prescribed Ceclor for an infection when he was five. Within minutes, Chuck developed a skin rash and swelling of the face, eyelids and joints. Our subsequent allergy tests showed that Chuck was indeed allergic to penicillin, and we concluded that he had a cross-sensitivity to cephalosporin. We recommended that for future bacterial infections Chuck be given erythromycin or sulpha drugs.

There are very few reports of allergic reactions to **erythro-mycin** in the medical literature, but in our Adverse Reaction Clinic we see a surprisingly large number of children who have reactions to this antibiotic. Symptoms include hives, joint pain and serum sickness and can occur either immediately after beginning treatment or several days later. Unfortunately, since little is known about the mechanism that causes erythromycin allergy, there aren't any good tests for determining the allergy.

Larry is a ten-year-old boy who was given erythromycin as treatment for a throat infection. After six days on the drug, he developed itchy hives all over his body, swelling of the lips, eyelids and face, swelling of the lymph glands in his neck, fever, and inflammation in his joints so severe that he found it painful to walk. We stopped the erythromycin and treated him initially with antihistamines. When that didn't help, we tried steroids. Although Larry's symptoms improved, it was several weeks before his rashes disappeared completely.

Allergic reactions to a fourth group of antibiotics, the **sulpha drugs**, can be similar—rashes or swelling of the face, lips and eyelids. Delayed reactions to sulpha can be more serious and involve the liver, kidney or brain. We have no tests to determine the early reactions to sulpha, but blood tests can detect susceptibility to a delayed reaction. Although sulpha allergy is less common than penicillin allergy, it is now showing up quite frequently in AIDS patients. When the drug is needed by these patients, we must use the desensitization technique (see page 159).

Multiple drug allergies

We have treated a few patients who seem to be allergic to all the common antibiotics. In each case, we take a detailed history of the type of reactions and when they occurred after each drug. We've noticed that a person with multiple drug allergies seems to have similar reactions to very different drugs, although we don't know why that is.

Sometimes there is a relationship between certain infectious diseases and drug allergies. For example, patients with infectious mononucleosis ("mono") are more likely to develop rashes when given penicillin. They also are more likely to have a positive skin test response to penicillin.

Allergic reactions in the operating room

Some people react to either general or local anaesthetic agents used in hospital, displaying symptoms ranging from very mild skin rashes to life-threatening collapse. That's why the anaesthetist always asks about allergies before an operation. If an allergy to a particular agent is suspected, the anaesthetist can use alternatives. If these aren't appropriate, various anti-allergic drugs can be given before and during surgery to block the reaction.

Doctors, nurses and hospital patients regularly exposed to rubber materials can have allergic reactions. For example, it is common to use rubber catheters in patients who have bladder problems. Doctors and nurses must wear rubber gloves in the operating room. The allergic symptoms are hives and worsening of eczema and, in extreme cases, life-threatening reactions a couple of hours into a surgical procedure. Fortunately, there are substitutes available for rubber, or anti-allergic drugs can be used before and during surgery.

Treatment of drug reactions

If you think you might be having a drug reaction, even if it is just a simple rash, stop taking the medication and call your doctor. The doctor will assess your symptoms and be able to tell you whether your symptoms are a normal side effect or a possible drug allergy. If there is only a mild rash, your doctor may want to continue you on the same drug. If the rash is extensive and also itchy, the drug will be stopped. You should then be referred to an allergist experienced in dealing with drug allergies.

To relieve the itching, your doctor may recommend an antihistamine or calamine lotion. If that doesn't help, or for more severe symptoms such as fever or arthritis, the doctor may prescribe a course of steroid therapy.

> **Any time you're having difficulty breathing as a possible drug reaction, have someone take you to the closest hospital.**

Any time you suspect a serious reaction, go to the hospital immediately. Take along your medication, so the medical staff will know what you've been taking and therefore can offer appropriate treatment.

ADVERSE REACTIONS TO VACCINES

Immunization has played a major role in halting the spread of many serious infectious diseases. Improved public health measures, better nutrition and antibiotics have also helped, but the success of vaccines is still remarkable. Smallpox has been wiped out world-wide, and other diseases such as diphtheria, measles, mumps, whooping cough (pertussis), polio and tetanus have been sharply curtailed in North America and other developed parts of the world.

Although there is a certain degree of risk associated with immunization, the benefits far outweigh the risks. The chance that you might suffer permanent illness or death from an infectious disease is much greater than the risk of a serious side effect from any of the vaccines used today. However, some people cannot be vaccinated in the normal way. At the Adverse Reaction Clinic in Toronto, we treat many patients who have had adverse reactions to vaccines. After a careful evaluation, we advise the patient as to the risks and benefits of continuing the course of vaccination. In certain cases, we administer tests to determine who might have a serious reaction to a particular vaccine, and then offer these people alternative methods for developing immunity.

Vaccines trigger the immune system

In Chapter 1, we defined allergy as an inappropriate or harmful response of the immune system. Vaccination, on the other hand, is a good example of the immune system working to protect the body against disease. The purpose of the vaccination is to trick your body into developing antibodies against certain infectious diseases, by exposing you to the disease.

Edward Jenner, a physician who lived in the late eighteenth century, originated vaccines. He recognized that milkmaids who contracted cowpox, a very mild illness that they caught from cows, never seemed to become ill with the more serious disease, smallpox. Jenner proved that by deliberately exposing people to cowpox, he could protect them from smallpox.

But the benefits of vaccination haven't come without some costs. One out of every fifty people immunized with Jenner's crude smallpox vaccine died. At the time, however, smallpox was so prevalent and treatment so crude that 40 per cent of the people who contracted the disease died. Thus the odds were better with the vaccine. The later, improved vaccines were much safer, but still one out of a million people vaccinated suffered brain damage. By the 1960's, vaccination protection was so common in the industrialized countries that the disease was rare. Then the small risk of a severe side effect outweighed the benefit of vaccination and the practice was stopped in North

America, except for international travellers. By 1979, smallpox had been eradicated world-wide and there was no longer a need for a smallpox vaccination.

Active immunization

For active immunization, we inject in the person either small doses of living but weakened organisms, which multiply in the body without causing disease, or purified components from killed viruses. The inoculated person then develops antibodies to this foreign substance. These antibodies will be ready to effectively fight off the real virus should that person later be exposed to it.

Recommended immunization schedule*

Age	Vaccine
2 months	DPT Polio[†] + Act-HIB[††]
4 months	DPT Polio + Act-HIB
6 months	DPT Polio + Act-HIB
after first birthday	MMR[†††]
18 months	DPT Polio + Act-HIB
4-6 years	DPT Polio
14-16 years	Td[††††] Polio
every 10 years thereafter	Td booster

[†]   DPT Polio means diphtheria, pertussis, tetanus and polio vaccine
[††]   Act-HIB means *Haemophilus influenzae* type B vaccine
[†††] MMR means measles, mumps and rubella vaccine
[††††] Td means tetanus and diphtheria

*Schedules may differ somewhat from province to province.

Usually a series of two or three shots is necessary to build up sufficient antibodies to provide long-lasting protection. To be effective, vaccination must be done before the person is exposed to the organism causing the disease, and therefore most immunization starts in the first year of life, as indicated in the chart on page 165.

The long-term memory of the immune system accounts for the success of many vaccines. Regular booster shots of some vaccines are necessary to maintain resistance to the disease. The booster reminds the immune system to keep producing protective antibodies.

Passive immunization

In emergency situations, pre-formed antibodies are injected to provide some temporary protection. This is necessary when a person hasn't maintained his immunity to tetanus with regular booster shots every ten years and then suddenly has an injury. We can also provide passive immunization against diseases we don't normally inoculate against, such as poisonous snakes or rabies.

Adverse reactions to routine immunization

Today, the vast majority of people can be immunized without problem. Some children and adults will experience minor side effects, such as a sore arm or a slight fever, but serious side effects are rare. When they do occur, however, they can cause permanent harm or be life-threatening.

The risk of serious side effects is often blown out of proportion in media reports. For example, between 1974 and 1978 there was so much publicity in the British papers about a few children who had developed neurological illnesses following a pertussis vaccination that the acceptance of pertussis vaccination dropped from 80 per cent to 31 per cent. As a result, there were two major pertussis epidemics in 1978.

But even though serious side effects are rare, we cannot become complacent about immunization. Vaccines consist of a mixture of active agents, antibiotics, preservatives, contaminating culture proteins and other additives. Any person who has had an adverse reaction to a particular vaccine should be evaluated by a doctor experienced in the field. The evaluation will include a detailed history and examination and, in certain cases, special skin tests of the components in the vaccine.

Diphtheria, pertussis and tetanus (DPT) vaccine

A routine series of DPT vaccinations can protect your child against three very serious illnesses:

- Diphtheria is an infection of the nose and throat that can interfere with breathing. It can cause heart failure and paralysis; one out of ten children who contract the disease dies from it.
- Pertussis, or whooping cough, is particularly serious in young children. They develop severe spells of coughing, which can interfere with eating, drinking and breathing; pneumonia commonly follows and many children develop convulsions or have severe brain damage. Some die from the disease.
- Tetanus, or lockjaw, is an infection usually resulting from a toxin or poison produced by the tetanus bacteria entering a wound. The muscles of the body go into spasm, and four out of every ten people with this disease die. It is now a rare condition because of the success of vaccination. The organism is still widespread in nature.

Before the DPT vaccine was available, these diseases were very common and caused many childhood deaths. Thus the benefit of protection outweighs the discomfort experienced by many infants following the DPT vaccination.

Reactions to DPT vaccine may be divided into two main groups—the adverse reactions and the allergy reactions. Minor adverse reactions are common and should not concern you unduly. These include a slight fever (under 40.5°C), redness or swelling at the site of inoculation, irritability, fretfulness, vomiting or diarrhea. If any of these symptoms occur or diarrhea lasts a few days, continue the vaccination course as planned. Be sure to tell your doctor, however, if symptoms are more severe. Hives, swelling of the eyelids or lips, breathing difficulties, limpness or a drop in blood pressure may be a sign of a rare allergy to the vaccine. This should be evaluated before proceeding with further shots.

After a DPT vaccination, tell your doctor if:

- your child's temperature goes above 40.5°C;
- crying lasts three or more hours or is unusually high-pitched;
- your child develops hives all over the body;
- there is swelling of the eyelids or lips.

If your child has breathing difficulties, convulsions or episodes of limpness, rush him immediately to a hospital emergency department.

Usually it is the pertussis component that causes adverse reactions. Thus, if appropriate, the doctor can eliminate pertussis from the vaccine used subsequently. This is often done for older children and adults, as pertussis is neither common nor severe past the age of seven.

Cathy had her first DPT shot at two months of age. Afterwards, she had a mild fever and was a bit cranky. Following her second shot at four months of age, she cried persistently for twenty-four hours, developed a fever and became pale and limp. Her doctor eliminated the pertussis component from the shot at six months of age and she didn't have any problems.

Although pertussis causes most adverse reactions, we occasionally treat a patient who is allergic to other components, such as the diphtheria vaccine.

Marie tolerated the first three shots of DPT with no adverse reactions. However, minutes after receiving a booster of DPT at eighteen months of age, she developed generalized hives, swelling of her lips and eyelids and breathing difficulties. She collapsed and needed an adrenaline injection and hospitalization for two or three days. Allergy tests showed that she was allergic to the diphtheria component.

To maintain immunity, you need boosters with tetanus and diphtheria (Td) vaccine every ten years throughout life. In order for Marie to maintain an adequate level of protection against diphtheria, she will need subsequent vaccinations administered in a special way. We will first desensitize her with very dilute doses of the vaccine. The dose will be gradually increased every fifteen minutes, as long as tolerated, until a normal dose is reached. We undertake this type of desensitization in hospital where we can use emergency measures immediately, if necessary.

Measles, mumps and rubella (MMR) vaccine
Before immunization with the MMR vaccine was available, hundreds of children died of pneumonia or inflammation of the brain, complications of red measles; others

became deaf or mentally retarded. One child in ten suffered temporarily from inflammation of the spinal cord and brain, a complication of mumps. Some adolescent boys and men who didn't contract mumps until they were sexually mature became sterile as a result of the disease infecting their testicles. Women who contracted rubella (German measles) while pregnant passed the infection on to their babies. As a result of the 1964 rubella epidemic in the United States, 25,000 children were born with heart defects, deafness, blindness or mental retardation. Other women who contracted rubella during pregnancy miscarried. Ninety per cent of children given one shot of MMR at twelve to fifteen months of age are protected for life, although when large outbreaks are expected, schools may require children be given a second dose of measles vaccine.

Some mild side effects of the MMR vaccine, such as a rash or slight fever five to twelve days after, and even a little swelling of the neck glands, occur in about one in five children. As well, a few children and adults receiving the MMR vaccine for the first time may experience temporary joint pain or numbness or tingling in their hands and feet. But these symptoms are minor when compared with the discomfort of even a mild case of one of these diseases. On rare occasions, more serious reactions do occur, but there is a much greater risk of problems occurring because of the diseases than as complications from the vaccine.

Since MMR vaccine is prepared by growing viruses on cells derived from chicken, we used to worry that children who were allergic to egg could have an allergic reaction to the MMR vaccine. But the MMR vaccine is prepared by growing viruses on chick cells, not egg embryos as with influenza virus.

Research at Johns Hopkins University in Baltimore has now shown that the vast majority of children allergic to egg will have no problem with MMR vaccine. Even children who have had a major anaphylactic reaction to egg have been successfully vaccinated with MMR. To be safe, however, any child who has had a life-threatening anaphylactic reaction to egg, with breathing problems, loss of consciousness or a fall in blood pressure, should be evaluated by an allergist prior to being given MMR. The doctor can confirm the egg allergy and can test for any possible reaction using skin tests with egg white and very dilute vaccine.

> **The measles, mumps and rubella vaccine contains trace amounts of neomycin. Therefore, a person who is allergic to neomycin may react when given the MMR vaccine.**

Despite the fact that most egg-allergic children are not in any danger from MMR vaccine, allergic reactions have occurred. This next case history demonstrates how something other than egg protein in a vaccine can cause such a reaction.

Nancy needed an MMR injection when she was seventeen years old because she didn't have adequate levels of the protective antibodies. Immediately, her blood pressure fell, she had difficulty breathing and she was rushed to hospital unconscious. There she was revived with adrenaline.

As we studied her history, we found that five years earlier she had been given neomycin for an eye infection. She had reacted with swelling and redness of the eyes—typical signs of a reaction to neomycin. She was not allergic to eggs.

Since the MMR vaccine may contain trace amounts of

neomycin, we concluded that Nancy was reacting to this drug in the vaccine.

Thus, it is important to tell your doctor about any food or drug allergies before vaccination.

Polio vaccine
Before the polio vaccine became widely available in the mid-1950's, hundreds of children died and many more were paralyzed by this virus. But now we can offer protection against polio in two ways. The most effective is the oral vaccine, which is given by mouth, usually in early infancy. Two or more doses in the first year, another at about eighteen months of age, and boosters when the child starts school and in the teenage years usually provide protection for life. The oral vaccine is an extract from the live viruses and, as such, very rarely causes paralysis, except in people who have a malfunctioning immune system.

Following vaccination, the live viruses survive for a time in the intestinal tract. Some of the viruses pass in the stool and can spread from the vaccinated person to other family members. Therefore, a child should not be given the oral polio vaccine if other family members are at risk of polio infection because they have cancer, leukemia or other diseases that damage the immune system. In some provinces, including Ontario, a killed vaccine is given in injectable form and as part of a combination vaccine to reduce the number of injections.

Haemophilus b vaccine
Haemophilus b vaccine provides protection against meningitis. There are no known allergies, although there are some reports of minor local reactions such as redness,

swelling and pain at the injection site, as well as mild fever.

Influenza vaccine

There are many viruses that cause influenza, or the flu. Each year scientists try to develop a vaccine that will help protect against the expected most common flu viruses. But flu shots are usually effective only for a season and protect against only one flu virus, not all. Thus, even if you have had flu shots, you may become ill. Flu shots are not given to everyone. The decision to protect against flu is a good example of balancing risk and benefit. Older people and people with heart and lung diseases are more likely to die from the flu, so they benefit most from the protection. Increasingly, annual flu shots are being recommended for younger people, including children with asthma or respiratory problems.

Anyone who is allergic to egg shouldn't have flu shots until skin testing is done as explained for the MMR vaccine, as this vaccine is developed from viruses grown on chicken embryos.

Other vaccines

To provide passive immunization for some problems, such as hepatitis, measles, poisonous snake bite and rabies, we can inject antibodies pooled from the blood of other people or animals who have developed the immunity. However, people with allergies to animal dander could have a severe reaction to the immunoglobulin used. These people should be allergy-tested with diluted vaccine before they are given the full dose.

There is also immunization available for certain diseases, such as typhoid, cholera and yellow fever, that are

Vaccine cautions

Despite the many benefits of vaccine protection, certain conditions bring an increased risk of serious side effects. Check with your doctor before allowing a vaccination for yourself or your child if the following conditions apply:

Vaccine	Conditions that increase risk of serious side effects
All vaccines	• any illness, other than a simple cold
MMR, yellow fever or influenza vaccine	• allergy to eggs
MMR vaccine	• allergy to antibiotics, such as neomycin
Live vaccines, such as Oral polio and MMR	• cancer, leukemia, lymphoma or any disease that lowers the body's resistance to infection
	• taking a drug that lowers the body's resistance to infection, such as cortisone or prednisone
All vaccines	• during pregnancy
All vaccines	• if there has ever been a serious reaction to previous inoculations

Also avoid oral polio vaccine if another family member has lowered resistance to infection, either because of disease or medication.

not common in North America but that you might encounter during travels to other countries. The yellow
fever vaccine also contains egg, so the same precautions
for people allergic to eggs apply as with the MMR vaccine
(see page 171).

CHAPTER NINE

Allergies to Insects

Practically everyone has experienced the unpleasant swelling, redness, itching and pain from insect bites and stings. Reactions such as these in the area of the bite are normal responses to the irritants and toxins in the saliva of biting insects and the venom from stinging insects.

Usually the swelling amounts to a small bump that appears within a few minutes and disappears in a few hours. Occasionally it may not be noticed for a day or two and can last for two to five days. Swelling from bites around the face, eyes and neck can become extremely large, even as large as a grapefruit, because the skin in these areas is quite loose. Rubbing the site tends to spread the swelling, and scratching a bite can cause infection in the area. Although large localized reactions can be frightening, you don't need special medical treatment, such as allergy shots. The chance that you'll have a more serious reaction the next time that type of insect bites or stings you is small—only about 5 to 10 per cent.

UNDERSTANDING INSECT ALLERGIES

Some people are very sensitive or allergic to venom from certain insects, particularly wasps and bees. They are likely to have a serious generalized reaction to a sting, involving other areas of the body such as the skin, stomach, throat, chest and heart.

Statisticians estimate that approximately forty to fifty people in North America die from insect stings each year, but this is probably an underestimation, as many may go unrecognized. Allergists would like to be able to predict who is likely to have a life-threatening generalized reaction, but that's impossible. As with allergies to drugs, we can't predict such insect allergies until you've been sensitized—that is, stung once.

Just because you have other allergies, you are not more at risk to insect allergy. Even in families where one member has had a severe reaction, other members may experience only localized reactions, and others no reaction at all.

Generalized reactions

Generalized reactions are rare, but they can be life-threatening. In one study, 187 factory workers were evaluated after insect bites and stings. Seventeen per cent had very large localized reactions, while only 4 per cent had significant severe reactions. Contrary to popular belief, allergic reactions to insects do not necessarily become worse with each subsequent sting. In fact, only about 5 to 10 per cent of people who have large localized reactions go on to a more severe generalized reaction. But since your doctor can't predict whether or not you'll be in that small group, he or she may recommend that, if you've had a large localized reaction, you carry one of the protective adrenaline kits described on page 182.

When they do occur, generalized allergic reactions usually begin within a few seconds to minutes after the bite, although they can be delayed up to an hour afterwards. As you can see from the list of symptoms in the box below, these are serious and, if treatment is not started soon enough, can result in death.

Symptoms of a generalized insect reaction

- a reddening of the skin over many parts of the body
- itchiness and hives over the entire body
- swelling of the eyelids, face, hands, lips or tongue
- stomach problems such as cramping, nausea, vomiting or diarrhea
- involuntary passage of urine
- swelling of the tongue and larynx (voice box) such that the person has trouble speaking
- laboured breathing
- rapid heartbeat
- lightheadedness or feelings of impending doom
- profuse sweating
- loss of consciousness or seizures

Sheryl experienced her first serious reaction to an insect sting while on a canoe trip through Algonquin Park to celebrate the completion of her final university exams. She was in the middle of Canoe Lake when a bee stung her on the arm. Within twenty minutes, her body was covered with hives; she found herself gasping for air and was quite faint. Her face, mouth and eyes were swollen and remained so for at least five hours. The next day she experienced similar but milder reactions, and over the next three days the reactions came and went.

Although it is possible, generalized reactions such as Sheryl's rarely lead to death the first time. Now that Sheryl is sensitized to the insect venom, however, there's a 50 to 60 per cent chance that she will have a similar, and possibly more severe, reaction to the next bite. If such a problem should again occur in a remote area, far from medical help, she would be in serious trouble. We therefore advised Sheryl to begin the following investigation and treatments.

Diagnosing an insect allergy

If you suspect that you or your child has an insect allergy, it should first be properly diagnosed. Since there is some risk associated with the testing, it should be done by an allergist who is experienced in this area and who can then start treatment, if necessary.

There are no reliable tests for allergies to mosquitoes or flies, but fortunately these insect bites are not as dangerous. It is the stinging insects that cause the generalized and more severe reactions in North America. These insects belong to the Hymenoptera family, and include the honeybee, wasp, yellow jacket, yellow hornet and white-faced hornet. An allergist can perform skin tests, as described in Chapter 2, for all of these insects. By using various concentrations, the doctor determines the degree of sensitivity and then decides on the best course of preventive treatment.

The blood RAST measurement, also described in Chapter 2, can determine whether you have a specific antibody to any of these stinging insects. However, it is expensive, it doesn't provide immediate results and it is not more sensitive than the skin test.

TREATMENT OF INSECT ALLERGIES

When a person who is allergic to insects is bitten, check first to see if there is a stinger in the skin. Honeybees leave behind barbed stingers that can continue to pump venom into the body. Using tweezers or your fingernails, remove the stinger immediately, being careful not to squeeze it in the process, as that will release more venom.

Treatment for localized reactions
To relieve the localized swelling and itching, you can use lotions, such as calamine lotion, and ice packs. Sometimes oral antihistamine medications, such as Benadryl, Chlor-Tripolon or Atarax, help reduce itching. It is important to try to avoid scratching, as that can lead to infection with its associated pain and fever.

Treatment for generalized reactions
If there are signs that this is a more serious reaction, you'll want to get medical help right away. But if you're off in the country, boating or hiking in an isolated area, you won't be able to wait. That's why a person who has an insect allergy should always have an emergency adrenaline kit close at hand during the spring, summer and fall months. Family members and friends should also learn how to use the kit in case you have difficulty administering the adrenaline yourself.

There are two such kits on the market. The Ana-Kit contains a pre-loaded adrenaline needle, an antihistamine and a tourniquet. The adrenaline effectively stops most serious reactions, and the antihistamine will help reduce the severity of reactions that may occur an hour or two later. You can use the tourniquet, but only for a few moments, if the bite is on the arm or leg to help reduce the spread of the venom through the blood stream.

The EpiPen Kit is particularly easy for non-medically trained teachers, baby-sitters or friends to use. The dose is regulated so that it is impossible to overdose or underdose. For children under the age of three, there is even an EpiPen Junior. Since the EpiPen Kit contains just the injectable adrenaline, you will need to carry some antihistamine tablets as well.

Whichever you or your doctor prefers, have several kits handy in the house, the cottage, the car, at school and at work. The instructions in the kits are very clear, but you should review these with your doctor before you need to use the adrenaline in an emergency situation.

Do not use adrenaline unless the person is having trouble breathing or feels faint. After you do use it, take the person immediately to a doctor's office or hospital emergency department.

It would be prudent for anyone with a history of life-threatening reactions to insects to also wear a Medic-Alert bracelet (see page 159).

Of course, the best strategy is to avoid contact with stinging insects when possible.

Eight-year-old Sarah lives on a farm where there are numerous insect nests. She has had many serious insect bites, and skin tests indicate that she is allergic to venom from yellow jackets. Removing all the insect nests from around Sarah's home is impossible, and her family can't move. Therefore we recommended that she always have an adrenaline kit close at hand, and that she build up her resistance to the venom with allergy shots.

Allergy shots (immunotherapy)

Although we've stated that we don't put much faith in allergy shots for hay fever (see page 75), we do use a form of immunotherapy, or desensitization, to help patients build up a tolerance to insects. It is a time-consuming, lengthy and expensive routine, so it is not recommended if the only reactions are itchiness or hives. Immunotherapy should only be used for people who have had a serious generalized reaction and have reacted positively to skin testing. Then it is worthwhile, as these people have a greater than 50 per cent chance of another life-threatening reaction.

Starting with very low doses, venom extract is injected weekly in gradually increasing amounts. Once the patient is receiving an amount of venom equal to that in two insect stings, the frequency of injections is cut back gradually to once every eight weeks. This form of therapy provides up to 95 per cent protection, but it must be continued for five years, or until the person no longer reacts positively to repeat skin and blood tests.

TYPES OF INSECTS

Both stinging insects and biting insects can cause adverse reactions. Allergic reactions to stinging insects are more severe; biting insects primarily cause local reactions.

Stinging insects

Stinging insects cause the most severe reactions in people with allergies. The five of special concern in North America all belong to the Hymenoptera family of insects. They are:

- honeybees
- yellow hornets
- white-faced hornets
- yellow jackets
- paper wasps

By learning a little about their habitats and habits, you will be better able to avoid them.

Honeybees have squat, hairy bodies with yellow and black markings. The wild bees live in hives in old trees, rock crevices or corners of houses and sheds; domesticated honeybees live in man-made hives. From early spring to late September, bees travel from their nests to gather nectar from nearby clover or honeysuckle plants. They tend to sting only when provoked or when you get in their way. If a bee comes near, remain calm and move away slowly; if it lands on you, brush it away gently. Swatting frightens the bee so that it is even more likely to sting. Bees die after stinging, but leave behind a stinger, so you'll be able to identify a bee sting.

Wasps and hornets are much more aggressive than bees and may sting repeatedly even when not provoked. They don't leave behind a stinger.

Both yellow and white-faced hornets nest in trees and shrubs and under the eaves of houses. Although their gray, paper-like nests are small, they are usually quite visible.

Yellow jackets have similar yellow and black markings to the bee, but their bodies are more elongated, like the hornet, although the yellow jackets are smaller. They tend to nest under logs or rocks or in small holes in the ground. Because of this, one of your best protections is to wear shoes and socks whenever you're walking outside.

Paper wasps nest under house eaves, on clothesline poles and in bushes. In the colder weather, they will take refuge in attics and closets and can be quite aggressive when discovered. Use caution when entering little-used areas of the house.

All these stinging insects are attracted to the odours of perfumes, cosmetics, hairspray, suntan lotion, fruit juices, soft drinks and beer. They also like the smell of certain paints. Their favourite colours are light yellow and blue, and they're also attracted by the heat from dark colours. At the present time, there aren't any repellents that effectively ward off stinging insects.

In the early spring, and periodically throughout the summer, have someone who does not have insect allergies inspect your home and garden for insect nests and remove them. Caution children not to throw stones or sticks at insect nests.

Call an exterminator to remove hornet nests. A local beekeeper may be willing to come to your property to relocate a bee colony. You may be able to knock down a wasp nest, but be sure to have someone spray it first with an insecticide to kill the wasps inside it.

Locate yellow jacket nests during the day, but wait until evening when the insects have returned to tackle them. Pour gasoline, kerosene or lye down the hole at least twice. The fumes will kill the insects; do not light the fuel.

Avoiding Stinging Insects

- Do not walk barefoot or wear open-toed sandals out-of-doors. Even hard beach sand can harbour certain types of wasps.
- Avoid using perfumes, hairsprays, hair tonics or other cosmetics, even scented soaps, which may attract insects.
- Stick to white, khaki or tan clothing, rather than bright or dark colours.
- Do not wear loose clothing or rough materials such as corduroy or denim in which insects may become trapped.
- Be careful when you shake out towels or clothing that have been left on the ground. Insects could be in the folds.
- Be careful when hiking, picnicking or camping. Insect repellents wear off and can't be relied upon to provide complete protection.
- Avoid orchards in bloom, clover fields and areas that are abundant with flowers.

Biting insects

Mosquitoes, fleas, black flies, deerflies, sandflies and ants primarily cause only local reactions when they bite. Rarely do these insects cause a more generalized or life-threatening problem. The itching is due to irritating substances from the insect's saliva. But if you rub or scratch the area, the swelling can spread and you could cause an infection.

Some insects found in the southern United States— the fire ant, harvester ant and kissing bug—have caused some more general reactions, as have deerflies and horse-

- Garden cautiously. Be well covered when mowing lawns, trimming hedges or pruning trees.
- Do not kick at rotting logs or bushes.
- Don't leave food outside uncovered. Never drink directly from a soft drink or beer can—there may be an insect inside.
- Store trash cans inside and keep the area clean. Spray insecticide around the cans periodically. Be watchful when handling the garbage.
- Look for insects before you get into a car. Drive with the windows closed. Also avoid riding horseback or on motorcycles or in convertible automobiles.
- Keep a cloth or can of insecticide handy in your car to trap or spray frightened insects. But don't panic. Generally the insect will fly out if you just open the window.
- If an insect approaches, stay still or move slowly. If it lands on you, do not slap it. Gently brush it away.

flies on occasion. Generalized reactions to biting insects are not a sign that you are likely to have problems with stinging insects.

Although there were a few testing materials available in the past, they were not reliable and have since been removed from the market. Desensitizing or allergy shots against these insects are not recommended, as it is difficult to obtain species-specific extracts and the reactions are not severe enough to warrant the procedure. The one exception is the fire ant, for which there are allergy shots.

The best strategy, then, is avoidance where possible. All the suggestions made for stinging insects apply (see page 186). If you do have troublesome bites, apply a cool compress, calamine lotion or steroid cream. Antihistamines may help reduce the swelling; if the site becomes infected, you may need an antibiotic.

CHAPTER TEN

Helping Allergic Children

We'd like to offer some final advice to parents, baby-sitters, grandparents and teachers. When you have a child with allergies, it can be disruptive for the entire family. You may have to buy and cook special foods; your family may not be able to have a dog or cat; you may have to do extra cleaning; or you may have to worry about insect stings every time you take a hike in the woods.

For your child, it may be even worse. Asthma attacks can be terrifying. Intense itching can interfere with sleep. Skin rashes can be embarrassing. And not being able to eat your friend's birthday cake seems downright unfair.

Allergies can interfere with all normal family activities and relationships, and even your work may be affected. Siblings may feel that one child is receiving most of the attention; parents may feel frustrated. If these feelings are allowed to run free, the emotional turmoil can become far more dangerous than the allergies themselves. As a parent of a child with allergies, you need to be constantly aware of how the disease is affecting your family dynamics, your child's self-esteem and the general quality of life in your family.

LEADING A NORMAL LIFE

The first thing you must do is stop blaming yourself. Sure, the tendency towards allergies is inherited, but so are your child's eye colour, merry smile and quick wit. It's all part of the gene package you give your children.

Don't blame your child, either, for the extra work allergies create. Your child may already be extremely uncomfortable and frightened. She doesn't want to burden you, but there's no alternative.

Having an allergic child may mean you're faced with extra demands. For example, if dust, smoke, animal dander or moulds are aggravating your child's health, changing your housekeeping procedures, as discussed in Chapter 5, can turn your home into a haven for your child. With advance planning, the extra work can be managed. In fact, if you throw dust collectors out before they add to the clutter, the house cleaning will be simplified.

Your baby may be covered with eczema, but underneath the skin she is an entirely healthy infant who needs cuddling and love. Doctors can provide medications to keep the eczema under control, but she also needs cuddling as reassurance of your love.

Learn as much as you can about the allergic problem. Certain consequences will be predictable, such as what happens when your child is stung by a bee. Reactions to foods may be less consistent, so you'll have to have your antennae out at all times, watching for possible risks. By understanding the action plan for management of the disease, you and your child can feel "in control."

With adequate preparation, a child with allergies can lead a normal life. She can go to camp, join the track team, learn to ride horseback and sleep over at a friend's house.

Don't become overprotective. When parents shield their children from all risks, they deny them opportunities to mature. Allow your child to take on increasing responsibility for the management of his disease as he grows. Help him to develop self-confidence.

Don't pamper your allergic child and she won't be inclined to become manipulative, demand special treatment or risk not taking her medication to attract attention. Give her the same amount of love and discipline that you give to all your children.

The less children with allergy diseases feel different from others, the better off they will be. With the newer methods of control, that is easier to achieve than in the past. See that your child benefits from medications that can lessen the severity and shorten the duration of the illness. In addition, peak flow meters can be used as early warning devices for asthma, and adrenaline kits can provide immediate response to insect stings and life-threatening food reactions.

Moving

Some families wonder whether a move to a different city might alleviate their problems. But there are no areas that are free of allergens. A person who has allergies in one part of the country is likely to develop allergies wherever she lives. It may, however, take four to six months for sensitization to occur, so you will probably not see symptoms at first. Only by living in an area will you find out how it affects your child.

Travelling

By taking a few precautions, you should be able to minimize vacation problems.

- Pack extra supplies of medications. You may need them when visiting a zoo, hiking in the country or staying in a cottage. If you're flying, be sure all medications are in your carry-on bag, not in the checked luggage.
- Children with frequent ear and nose complications may need extra medication to help tolerate pressure changes during take-off and landing. Ask your doctor to prescribe the appropriate medication.
- Some airlines now have a no-smoking policy, even on longer flights. Check when making your arrangements.
- Before car trips, be sure the car is clean and the air filters are working. Air conditioning can help in maintaining the air quality. There should be no smoking in the car.
- Check on the locations of hospitals or emergency clinics in your destination city. Know where you can go for help so you don't become flustered in an emergency.

School

Once a child enters school, there will be a host of new problems. You can no longer control your child's environment or activity pattern; children with food allergies may exchange foods with other children; children with asthma encounter chemical smells, smoke, dust, moulds and pollens at school. If asthma is poorly controlled, exercise or cold air at recess time may be a problem.

Although school-aged children are not as likely to require hospitalization for their allergies, they may miss school often, and even when they are in school they may not be functioning optimally. If asthma or eczema is disrupting their sleep, they won't be able to function as well the next day in school. With modern medicines, asthma can be brought under control, and these children will be able to thrive in school.

On occasion, you may have to run interference for your child with school personnel. Teachers may not really believe him when he says he can't go out for recess on a certain day. They may even accuse him of bringing on an asthma attack to obtain attention. If children are dealt with honestly and are allowed to participate fully in classroom activities, they develop self-confidence. They need not feel different or less capable because they are allergic.

Parents have an obligation to tell teachers about their children's health problems in a frank and open manner. The days of hiding diseases are over. Children who have allergic problems such as stuffy noses, asthma or eczema may be affected in very subtle ways by changes in weather, exposure to dust or viral infections. Fatigue, lack of concentration and irritability may be the only signs of problems. Because of this, teachers and parents should alert each other when children regularly or even unexpectedly show these signs. The more you prepare teachers and caregivers in advance, the better.

We do not expect teachers and other school personnel to become doctors or nurses. They cannot know all the details of the various illnesses their students have. However, open communication between teachers, patients

Teachers can help children with asthma

- Do not regard children with asthma as lazy if they must restrict their participation in exercise or sports. Don't embarrass them. Encourage rather than discourage their participation, but don't allow them to ignore their symptoms. Teenagers, especially, may deny problems in order to continue playing.

- Permit children with asthma to stay indoors at recess when the temperature is extremely cold. Extreme temperature changes are likely to aggravate an asthmatic condition, especially when combined with exercise.

- If recommended by their doctor, allow children to use an inhaler fifteen to twenty minutes before gym class or when having attacks.

- School policies restricting the possession of medication by students are often inappropriate. Allow students with sufficient maturity to carry their medications at all times so that there is no unnecessary delay when it is needed.

and parents is essential to help maintain appropriate management regimens.

Teenagers

Older children and adolescents often become discouraged with a chronic disease. They want to get on with their life, without the hassle of regular medication. They are notorious risk-takers; they test the limits of their disease; they neglect to take their medication; and they may begin to smoke—both ordinary cigarettes and mari-

It does not help a child having an asthma attack in a far corner of a playground if his medication is locked somewhere in the school.

- If students are found overusing their inhalers, this is usually a sign that they require more and different medications. In this situation, parents should be informed of these occurrences so they can seek further medical help.

- At every school, some staff members should have completed cardiopulmonary resuscitation (CPR) and basic first aid training. They should also know how to use injectable forms of adrenaline, such as EpiPens, and these should be available in several locations in the school. It is virtually impossible to overdose or cause significant harm to anyone with the single measured dose available from these units. They can be life-saving in cases of serious bee stings in the school playground or if a child accidentally eats something he is allergic to, such as peanuts.

juana. All of this can have an extremely adverse effect on them if they are asthmatic. In fact, a child who may seem to have outgrown asthma can have it reoccur if he or she begins smoking.

Often we find that a teenager who is thought to have outgrown asthma still has extensive symptoms of the disease but has learned to tolerate them. When these teens have lung function tests, it can be quite surprising how low their lung capacity is. Yet they are not complaining about asthma. They do not know what it is to be normal.

Complacency is a natural way of dealing with problems, but it can be dangerous with asthma. Teenagers and young adults will often underestimate the nature of their disease and try to ignore it. But by ignoring their disease, they increase the risk of having a severe, life-threatening episode, and no one else realizes the seriousness of the situation.

Several years ago, we were treating a teenage girl who had an allergy to peanut. One day she accidently ate a chocolate bar that contained peanuts. She knew immediately that she was having a reaction, but since previous reactions had been relatively mild, she chose to wait it out. This time she developed swelling in her bronchial tubes that blocked her breathing. By the time the ambulance came, it was too late.

As happens after any such death, her parents were both angry and full of guilt. Could they have done anything to prevent this tragedy? Even with medical treatment close at hand, allergy deaths do occur if that treatment is not used soon enough or aggressively enough. Children have not died during asthma attacks because of overuse of medication. If anything, it has been the lack of recognition and undertreatment of asthma that has led to unexpected deaths.

Open communication
The way to prevent small problems from becoming major issues is with open communication—with all your children, their friends, their teachers, counsellors and baby-sitters, and with your doctor.

Each patient, along with his parents, caregivers and close friends, must understand what signs and symptoms are part of the illness pattern, and what to do in response—that is, whether to take certain medications or simply to communicate concerns.

When issues arise or if you feel frustrated, talk to your doctor. The problems you are facing are common. Chances are he or she has helped some other family deal with them before.

The new scientific research into the immune system and the mechanisms involved in allergic responses has already helped us improve our treatment strategies. Allergy sufferers can expect even better treatment as doctors learn better ways to manipulate the immune system, as we improve our ability to institute avoidance of allergens and environmental changes, as drug companies develop safer and more effective drugs, and as doctors and patients learn to recognize allergies, asthma and rhinitis diseases that respond best to early, appropriate medical treatment. We are confident that, in the future, allergy patients will experience fewer problems and complications.

HOW TO ADMINISTER EPINEPHRINE

Immediate use of epinephrine (adrenaline) at the time of a life-threatening reaction to insect bites and stings, foods, drugs and exercise-induced anaphylaxis can save a life. It is the only drug to use in this way.

- Don't be afraid to administer epinephrine, in the form of a spring-loaded EpiPen or a preloaded syringe (Ana-Kit).

- Administer epinephrine as early as possible after the onset of a severe reaction. Both EpiPen and Ana-Kit come with easy-to-follow instructions for administering an injection directly into the outer thigh muscle. After removing the safety cap, the EpiPen can be injected immediately. Once the needle is jabbed in, hold it in place for a few seconds after the unit activates. With the Ana-Kit, you must first hold the syringe upright and push plunger to expel air; then rotate the plunger 1/4 turn to the right until it aligns with a slot in the barrel of the syringe. After the needle is inserted, push the plunger until it stops to deliver a full adult dose.

- After an injection, rush the person to a nearby hospital emergency department for continued observation as there may be a delayed reaction.

- One injection is usually enough, but if breathing is still laboured or the person becomes unconscious, a second dose can be given after 15 or 20 minutes.

- Adult supervision is mandatory at this time as a person can become disoriented during a reaction.

- Epinephrine must be readily available, not locked in drawers or cupboards. All school staff should be aware of its location.

- Children old enough to understand its use should be allowed to carry their own epinephrine devices. Multiple devices should be available as backup in various areas of their school.

Glossary

Allergen   A common substance, usually a protein, that starts an allergy response.

Allergist   A medical doctor with additional specialized training in the treatment of allergic and other similar diseases.

Allergy   An inappropriate or harmful response by the immune system to a normally harmless substance.

Anaphylaxis   A life-threatening allergy reaction that involves many organs of the body. The muscles around the airways may go into spasm, making it difficult to breathe; blood vessels expand rapidly causing a sudden drop in blood pressure, which may lead to unconsciousness and death.

Angioedema   Widespread swelling of the deeper layers of the skin.

Antibody   A protein formed by certain white blood cells that responds to specific foreign particles when they enter the body. Immunoglobulin E (IgE) is one kind of antibody that recognizes allergens when they enter the body.

Antigen Any foreign substance not normally present in the body which, when introduced into the body, stimulates the production of antibodies. Allergens are one group of antigens.

Antihistamine A drug that relieves some allergy symptoms by chemically blocking the action of histamine.

Anti-inflammatory medications Sprays, liquids and pills that reduce the swelling and other features of inflammation and thus relieve many symptoms of allergies and asthma.

ASA (acetylsalicylic acid) An ingredient in many pain-killers (e.g., Aspirin) and some arthritis drugs.

Asthma Difficulty in breathing because the airways are narrowed due to inflammation and spasm of the muscles around the airways. The hallmark symptoms are wheezing, coughing and shortness of breath at night, in the early morning or with exercise.

Atopic person An atopic person is a person who has allergies. The immune system of an atopic person produces greater than normal amounts of IgE antibodies.

Basophil cells Cells in the blood that release chemicals during an allergy reaction.

Bronchial tubes The tubes through which air passes from your nose and mouth into your lungs, and back out again.

Bronchitis An infection of the airways.

Bronchodilators Inhaled medications that relax the muscles surrounding the bronchial tubes, making it easier for a person with asthma to breathe.

Bronchospasm   Contraction of the muscles lining the airways, thus narrowing the passage.

Challenge testing (oral)   A method of testing for food allergies. A very small amount of food is eaten and symptoms are watched for. In an "open" challenge the person knows when the food is being tried; in a "blind" challenge the food is disguised.

Chestiness   Laboured breathing, wheezing or a rattling noise in the chest.

Chronic   Something that happens regularly over a long period of time.

Conjunctivitis   Inflammation or infection of the eyes with swelling, itching, redness and watering.

Coughing   A reflex action of the chest and diaphragm muscles that forces air quickly out of the breathing tubes.

Dander   Skin scales from an animal, a common allergen.

Decongestant   A medication that reduces congestion, usually used to relieve the congestion in the nose that accompanies rhinitis or colds.

Dust mite   An extremely small insect that lives on dead skin scales and is found in house dust.

Eczema   Red, itchy patches on the skin that can be either dry and flaky or wet and weepy. Eczema can be an allergic response (atopic eczema), but not all eczema is caused by allergies.

Hay fever   More correctly called allergic rhinitis. Refers to the itching, swelling, congestion and discharge from the nose produced by allergens.

Histamine   One of the mediators, a chemical released from mast cells when they have been activated by an allergen.

Hives   Itchy skin rash with white raised areas or wheals surrounded by redness. Sometimes hives look like a cluster of mosquito bites; sometimes they resemble large welts.

IgE antibody   Immunoglobulin E antibody is one type of antibody that recognizes allergy-causing substances when they enter the body.

Immune system   A mechanism by which your body fights off infection or invasion by foreign materials. It involves specialized cells containing specific chemicals. In an atopic person, the immune system kicks into action when some harmless substances enter the body.

Immunoglobulin   A type of protein. Immunoglobulin E (IgE) is the particular antibody that is produced in greater than normal quantities in a person with allergies.

Immunotherapy   A series of injections containing known allergens. Commonly referred to as allergy shots.

Inflammation   Swelling, redness and heat in certain body tissues as a result of fluids leaking into the tissue from the blood vessels. Inflammation in tissues is the cause of many of the problems associated with allergic disease.

Inhalant allergens   Substances in the air, such as dust, pollens, animal dander, moulds and fungal spores that can cause allergic reactions.

Irritant   Anything that may irritate or worsen inflammation in the tissues. Cold air can be an irritant for a person with asthma.

Late response inflammation   Inflammation that occurs several hours after exposure to an allergen. This inflammation is more generalized and lasts much longer than the initial allergy response.

Lymphocytes   Specialized white blood cells that participate in immune and allergy responses. They are of two major types, T cells, which control many immunologic responses and B cells, which produce antibodies that recognize invading foreign particles.

Macrophages   Large white blood cells that act as scavengers. They engulf microorganisms and antigens. In the immune response they present the antigen to T lymphocytes in a special way that allows the T lymphocyte to recognize it as foreign.

Mast cells   Cells in mucosal tissues that release chemicals, called mediators, that begin the chain of events associated with an allergic reaction.

Mediators   Potent chemicals released from activated mast cells that cause the symptoms of allergic disease. Histamine is one such mediator.

Mucosal tissue   The layer of body cells that lies just below the surface of the skin. A mucous membrane also lines the respiratory tract (nose and lungs) and the digestive tract. This is where allergy reactions occur initially.

Mucus   Phlegm or discharge from any mucosal tissue.

Peak flow meter   A device that measures the rate at which a person can expel air from his lungs. The device measures the rate of airflow in litres per minute. When the bronchial tubes are inflamed, the rate of airflow is much slower than normal. Thus this device can signal an early warning that the bronchial tubes are becoming inflamed.

Perennial   Something that occurs throughout the year.

Pollen   The male sex cells of trees, grass and weeds. Pollen is carried by the wind and on animals so that the plant can reproduce in a new location.

Radio-allergosorbent test (RAST)   A type of blood test that measures the level of IgE antibodies in your bloodstream to a particular allergen.

Rhinitis   Inflammation in the nose with associated symptoms of itching, congestion and clear discharge. Commonly but incorrectly called hay fever.

Seasonal   Something that occurs only at certain times of the year.

Sensitization   The initial response to an allergen that results in the production of specific IgE antibodies.

Serum sickness   A complex of symptoms, including rashes, fever, swelling of the face, eyelids or lips, puffiness in the hands and feet, and arthritis or pain in the joints.

Symptom   Bodily changes that are not normal; a sign that something is wrong.

Urticaria   A medical term for hives.

Wheezing   A whistling sound heard when a person is having difficulty breathing out through narrowed bronchial tubes. A hallmark of asthma.

Useful Addresses

Allergy and Asthma Information Association
Suite 750
30 Eglinton Avenue West
Mississauga, Ontario L5R 3E7
(905) 712-2242

The AAIA is a national organization of more than 5,000 members—people with allergies and interested health professionals. There are regional offices in Vancouver, Edmonton, Scarborough, Montreal and New Brunswick and chapters across Canada. AAIA receives approximately 18,000 inquiries about allergies per year. For a $35.00 annual fee, members receive a quarterly newsletter. Fact sheets and special cookbooks are also available.

The Canadian Dietetic Association
Suite 601
480 University Avenue
Toronto, Ontario M5G 1V2
(416) 596-0857

Call to ensure that the dietitian or nutritionist who is

giving you advice is a member of this association. Membership ensures that the person has a recognized university degree in foods and nutrition and has completed a dietetic internship.

Canadian Medic-Alert Foundation
P.O. Box 9800, Station A
Don Mills, Ontario M3C 2T9
(416) 696-0267

Call or write for an application form. The membership fee of $30.50 (payable by Mastercard, VISA, cheque or money order) covers the cost of a Medic-Alert bracelet and a wallet card. These provide health professionals with key information about your allergies, should there ever be an emergency in which you could not speak for yourself.

Food Allergy Network
4744 Holly Avenue
Fairfax, VA, USA 22030-5647
(703) 691-3179

The Food Allergy Network has a number of publications, a regular newsletter and laminated wallet-size cards with useful information on reading food labels.

Index